Quality Assurance
in Medical Education

Geraldine MacCarrick

Quality Assurance in Medical Education

A Practical Guide

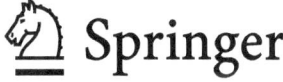 Springer

Geraldine MacCarrick
School of Medicine and Dentistry
James Cook University
Cairns Clinical School
Cairns
Queensland
Australia

ISBN 978-0-85729-712-9   ISBN 978-0-85729-713-6   (eBook)
DOI 10.1007/978-0-85729-713-6
Springer London Heidelberg New York Dordrecht

Library of Congress Control Number: 2012944641

Printed on acid-free paper

Springer is part of Springer Science+Business Media (www.springer.com)

*To Terry for his ideas, support, and encouragement
to the end.
To Róisín for her smiles and harp music
throughout the writing.
Chun Don agus Deirdre as a dtacaíocht agus grá.*

Preface

Preparing a medical school or postgraduate medical education program for accreditation or review is a challenging process requiring a clear understanding of the standards being used, sufficient resources, and adequate preparation and planning. As a medical educationalist involved in curriculum reform in both hemispheres, it has become apparent that continual change and renewal are part of the shifting landscape in which we operate. Such change however needs to occur within the context of agreed educational standards. Familiarity and compliance with such standards is now a necessary part of medical program leadership. The process of accreditation should be viewed by medical education leaders, not as a threat, but as an opportunity to continue to drive the quality improvement agenda.

Geraldine MacCarrick
BMedSc(Hons)MBBS, DTM, MPH,
MBA, FRACGP, FRACMA, PhD

Contents

Chapter 1
Getting Underway

Introduction

Most medical education institutions across the globe come under regular review and accreditation by national and/or regional bodies. Well-known examples include the Australian Medical Council (AMC) in Australia, the General Medical Council (GMC) in the UK, and the Liaison Committee on Medical Education (LCME) in the USA. Preparing a medical institution for institutional review or accreditation can be challenging, requiring an understanding of the international standards being used, adequate resources, preparation, and planning. This book provides a practical guide for medical educators preparing their medical education program for independent review. Use of internationally accepted standards and how these standards "drive" the quality improvement agenda in medical education are described.

Commitment to any self-review process requires top level support from within the medical education institution. Once the decision is taken to conduct a review of the medical education program, either as part of a continuous cycle of self-review or in preparation for accreditation, dedicated resources need to be identified to support the activity. Usually, this is achieved using a project management approach (see Fig. 1.1).

G. MacCarrick, *Quality Assurance in Medical Education,*
DOI 10.1007/978-0-85729-713-6_1,
© Springer-Verlag London 2013

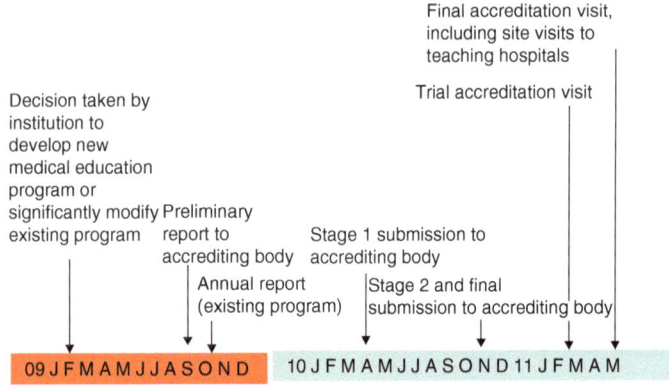

FIGURE 1.1 Example timeline from decision to introduce or significantly modify medical education program to accreditation

A comprehensive communication strategy to accompany the project will facilitate engagement of faculty and students and key external stakeholders. Important stakeholders include regulatory bodies such as medical councils, specialist colleges, teaching hospitals, and medical associations. A dedicated newsletter and website can provide a useful adjunct to such a strategy, providing regular progress reports on the key priority areas for improvement in the lead-up to an external review.

Context and Change in Medical Education

Understanding the context in which the institution is operating is an important consideration prior to preparing for an external accreditation or review. Typically, most medical education programs will be undergoing some form of continuous improvement at the time of a proposed quality assurance visit. The institution itself may be undergoing governance restructure, for example, away from a traditional discipline-based structure toward greater integration of teaching and learning. Such reforms need to be carefully communicated and understood by faculty and students. In addition, faculty and students need to understand the rationale and significance of a proposed external review and what contribution is expected from them. An external review can present the institution with a valuable opportunity to "drive" the quality improvement agenda.

It is advisable for those responsible for leading reform to be familiar with the literature on change management and the factors associated with implementing successful reform in the medical education setting. Change itself affects every aspect of an educational organization whether it is incremental change (targeting refinements such as introducing a new module or a new form of teaching delivery) or more fundamental reform such as moving wholesale to an "outcomes-focused" curriculum. The context in which the institution is operating will impact on the timing and possibly success of an externally led quality assurance process. Familiarity with some of the known barriers to reform in medical education can inform the changes which the institution is proposing and the approach taken.

Barriers to Change in Medical Education

Large-scale coherent medical education reform has proven a difficult task in many countries. Cuban reported a mere 5 % of medical institutions studied had embraced fundamental change – that is, had radically reformed their curricula from the traditional Flexner model to a more integrated curriculum [1]. The Association of American Medical Colleges [2] previously identified five specific barriers to change: faculty members' inertia, lack of leadership, lack of oversight of the educational program, limited resources, and lack of evidence that implementing the change would result in the necessary improvements. It has also been shown that the culture of each medical institution influences critical elements such as educational philosophy, leadership, and resources and shapes the type of change that results [3]. Most of the barriers to change in medical education which the literature identifies relate to the ways in which medical institutions are governed and funded and how these can potentially prevent improved coordination of the medical education process.

Coordination of Quality Assurance Process

Having taken the decision to prepare for an externally led quality assurance review, it is advisable to appoint a dedicated team or department with intimate knowledge of the institution's curriculum and governance to coordinate the effort. Such a team will require sufficient delegated authority to ensure cooperation from all faculty. Typically, this is the remit of the institution's Department of Medical Education. Such departments are variously called Medical Education Units, Centre for Educational Research, Centre for Medical and Health Science Education, or Centre for Educational Development and have become almost an essential requirement for a medical training establishment [4].

The functions of such departments include research, teaching, and support of academic staff (see Fig. 1.2). Typically, such departments are familiar with the entire curriculum and how it is delivered and have oversight of the faculty development program. Medical education units are usually associated with the medical institution executive office, for example, the Dean's office. In the case of the medical school, close communication with a supportive dean is an essential part of successful preparation for an accreditation visit. The elements of successful leadership of the Department of Medical Education have been described [4]:

> He/she should be in a position to foster scholarly habits among the staff... have a flair for teaching... a reputation for innovation... can convey a sense of excitement about teaching... sets a challenging climate for academic work and stimulates the lively exchange of ideas between colleagues (p. 671).

Davis and colleagues also point out the need for the Medical Education Unit to be closely integrated with the faculty and not seen as a separate entity. Such a department is well placed to coordinate the communication strategy and define the key milestones ahead in preparation for accreditation.

Regular curriculum "away days" or retreats are a useful way to update on new innovation and proposed reforms and also useful in the lead-up to an accreditation visit.

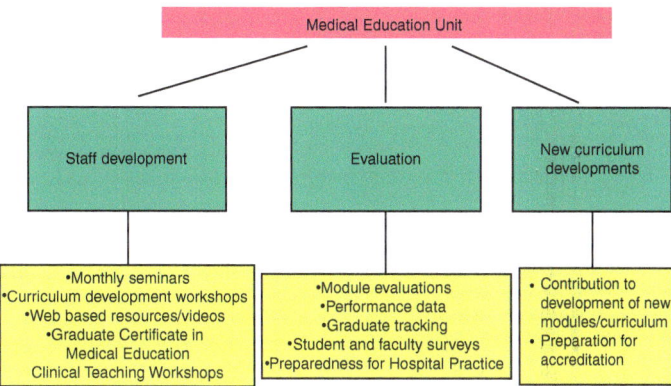

FIGURE 1.2 Typical activities of a Department of Medical Education

A theme for such events can be those areas of the medical education program which are likely to come under review by the accrediting team, such as aspects of the program that have changed since previous reviews. Figure 1.3 shows an excerpt from a typical annual curriculum retreat. If the proposed accreditation visit represents a "high-stakes" assessment of the program, some institutions schedule a "trial" accreditation visit in preparation for the actual visit (see above timeline). In such a case, it is advisable to select "mock" external assessors who are both familiar with the standards used and are recognized experts in their discipline.

The Accrediting Team

Site visits conducted by visiting teams are the main means by which most medical education programs are reviewed against the relevant accrediting body's standards and against the institution's own defined goals and objectives. The team is responsible for preparing a report that identifies strengths and areas for improvement. Typically, the accrediting body advises the

Purpose of the Forum is to...
- Provide an opportunity to reflect on progress made against annual "road map"
- Identify ongoing areas of threat/weakness and workshop means of addressing these prior to proposed accreditation visit
- Communicate new curriculum developments since last Forum

Time	Session	Presenters/facilitators	
11:30–11:45	Curriculum governance • Curriculum & assessment board, the cycle directors and faculty executive	Dean & Chair of curriculum & assessment board	Background papers for inclusion in pre-reading pack:
11:45–12:00	Curriculum outcomes • Curriculum mission and medical graduate profile	Vice Dean Medical Education and Chair of Curriculum Outcomes Working Group	• Rationale for curriculum renewal and accreditation • Curriculum governance • Road map...progress so far • Report of Curriculum Outcomes Working Group
12:00–12:15	• Curriculum database		• New curriculum assessment strategy
12:15–12:30	• Assessing curriculum outcomes	Vice Dean Junior Cycle and Chair of Assessment Working Group	• The five themes of the medical curriculum
12:30–12:45	Q & A Session		
12:45–1:30pm	Focus: Embedding the five curriculum themes vertically and horizontally	Five theme champions	

FIGURE 1.3 Curriculum retreat

institution in writing about the timing of the assessment, the process that will be undertaken, and the documentation required. This initial contact is typically 1 year in advance. The visit is agreed in consultation with the head of the institution. A visit typically lasts about 1 week. It is important to recognize that the institution's written submission to the accreditation team forms the basis for the visit. Most accreditation bodies will outline the specific requirements for this documentation. For example, it may be necessary to submit detailed plans for future capital development of the institution if this is proposed or areas may be identified by the accrediting team based on previous site visits as warranting particular attention. It is essential to liaise closely with the accrediting team over the content of the written submission. In the case of a follow-up visit, the report will likely focus on those areas that have changed *since* the last visit. Some accrediting bodies will also invite a separate submission from the medical students' association. All written submissions to the accrediting body are usually invited at least 4 months before the on-site visit to allow the accrediting team to read carefully the documentation and request additional clarification if required.

The visiting teams will typically have an appointed team leader; members with extensive medical education experience, medical student representation and, in the case of the General Medical Council (UK), lay members are invited to participate. Other members may include medical specialists, specialty trainees, experienced academic, and health service managers. The group composition will reflect the areas the team wishes to focus on. In addition, the composition of the team should provide for a balance of assessors from different medical institutions, the basic and clinical disciplines, hospital and community-based teachers, community interest groups, and gender balance. The size of the team will depend on the areas of focus for the review but will typically number about six members and a team leader. The chair has overall responsibility for the conduct of the assessment. The accrediting body will typically provide secretariat support. The role of the secretariat is to provide policy advice and collate and edit the team's report.

Typically, the assessment team will hold a preliminary team meeting several months before the site visit, during which the team identifies key issues it will focus during the visit. The teams focus is informed by the institution's written submission and previous institution reports. During this preliminary meeting, the outline schedule for the visit is prepared for future discussion with the head of the institution. Any further information which the team needs can be requested after this meeting.

The program for the visit is agreed in advance between the head of school/program and the visiting team. During the week-long visit, the team will aim to meet as many heads of department as possible as well as hospital teaching staff; the curriculum committee; committees in medical education and research; representative academic staff, recent graduates, and students (see Fig. 1.4). In the case of a medical school accreditation, the team may also consult with senior University appointments and representatives of the local departments of health and the agency responsible for intern training. The program for the visit should aim to provide adequate opportunity for discussion with staff and students from as many training sites as possible as well as external stakeholders. Meetings with students/trainees are conducted privately, that is, in the absence of faculty, and maintaining anonymity and confidentiality is an important consideration. Following the visit, the assessment team prepares a formal report which is used to make recommendations regarding accreditation and to provide feedback to the institution. As it often takes several weeks before a final report is compiled, some quality assurance teams provide a verbal summary statement at the conclusion of the visit. While these preliminary comments are not binding, they are nonetheless a useful source of immediate feedback to staff and students and are usually well received, particularly given the significant investment of effort required to prepare for an external review. Once a final decision is reached with respect to accreditation, the accrediting body will formally notify the program executive and other relevant authorities (e.g., the university, the college, the medical boards, and the Medical Council) of the decision. A summary of the final report is usually available as a public document.

Standards Used

Most of the accrediting bodies use a set of standards against which they accredit their medical education programs. Most of the standards used are closely aligned with the standards articulated by the World Federation for Medical Education (WFME). The Executive Council of the WFME first published a position paper on the topic of international standards in medical education in 1998. Subsequently, an international

Time & venue	Session title	Main presenter
8:00–8:15	Morning briefing with the Dean	Dean and Visiting Team Chair
1. Regional hospital (Team members A,B & C)		
9:30–10:00	**Tour of facilities**	
10:00–10:30 10:30–11:30	Meeting with Professor of Surgery Meeting with Professor of Medicine	
11:30–12:00	Meeting with CEO, Regional Hospital	
11:00–12:00	Lunch Meeting with Chair of Medical Executive Regional Hospital Divisional Directors, Nurse Co-Directors Clinical Teachers Intern Coordinators	
2. Rural hospital (Team members D,E,F)		
9:30–10:00	**Tour of facilities**	
10:00–10:30 10:30–11:30	Meeting with Professor of Medicine Meeting with Professor of Surgery	
11:30–12:00	Meeting with CEO, Rural Hospital	
11:00–12:00	Meeting with Director Medical Services and Divisional Directors, Nurse Co-Directors Clinical Teachers Intern Coordinators	
1:30–3:00	**Group Tour of Clinical Laboratory**	
2:00–3:00 3:00–5:00	Program Evaluation Results Meeting with Senior Students	Chair, Evaluation Working Group

FIGURE 1.4 Example itinerary for medical school accreditation visit

task force was established with the purpose of defining international standards for basic [undergraduate] and postgraduate medical educational programs. The main purpose of the task force was to develop medical education standards that could be applied internationally. Key considerations in developing the WFME standards were that the standards should serve as an impetus for institutional self-evaluation and that the standards should take full account of the many different approaches to medical education in different countries. It was specifically intended that the standards should *not* dictate content or inhibit educational innovation and that the standards should *not* be used to rank institutions:

> The primary intention of WFME in introducing an instrument for quality improvement is to provide a new framework against which medical institutions can measure themselves in voluntary institutional self-evaluation and self-improvement processes [5].

It was acknowledged however that the standards might be used as part of a system for national or international accreditation of medical education programs [6]. The standards have since been informed by and further refined based on feedback from international advisors and from a number of conferences around the world. The WFME standards for medical education are structured under nine key headings including the mission of the institution, the education/training program itself, the assessment of students/trainees, support for students/trainees, teaching and supervising staff, educational resources to support teaching, program evaluation, and how the medical education program is governed. In the UK, the General Medical Council (GMC) Quality Improvement Framework for Undergraduate and Postgraduate Medical Education and Training in the UK sets out how the GMC will quality assure medical education and training in the UK. The standards and outcomes used are those set out in Tomorrow's Doctors [7] and The Trainee Doctor [8]. The GMC standards are also grouped broadly under domains including patient safety; student selection; design and delivery of the curriculum; assessment; support and development of students, teachers, and the local faculty; management of the curriculum; resources; capacity; and outcomes. In the USA and Canada, the Liaison Committee on Medical Education (LCME) [9] accredits medical education programs which are operated by universities or medical institutions that are chartered in the USA or Canada. Accreditation of Canadian medical education programs is undertaken in cooperation with the Committee on the Accreditation of Canadian Medical Institutions. To achieve and maintain accreditation, a medical education program leading to the M.D. degree in the USA and Canada must meet the standards described by the LCME. The LCME standards are organized around the following five headings including the institutional setting (i.e., governance and academic environment), the educational program (including objectives, structure, design, and content), students, faculty, and resources.

Summary Points

- Preparing a medical education program for review or accreditation requires an understanding of the international standards being used and adequate preparation and planning.
- Preparation includes a communication strategy. Staff, students, trainees, and other stakeholders need to understand the rationale and significance of the quality assurance process including what is to take place and their contribution.
- Institutions and accrediting teams should work cooperatively meeting agreed deadlines for written submissions and providing additional information as requested.
- The program for the visit should aim to provide adequate opportunity for face-to-face discussion with staff and students from as many training sites as possible.
- Annual staff retreats are a particularly useful way to update staff in the lead-up to an accreditation visit.
- External review can present the institution with the impetus to "drive" the quality improvement agenda.

References

1. Cuban L. Change without reform: the case of Stanford University School of Medicine, 1908–1990. Am Educ Res J. 1997;34(1):83–122.
2. Association of American Medical Colleges. Physicians for the twenty-first century. The GPEP report: report of the Panel on the General Professional Education of the Physician and College Preparation for Medicine. Washington D.C.: Association of American Medical Colleges; 1984.

3. Cohen J, Dannefer EF, Seidel HM, Weisman CS, Wexler P, Brown TM, et al. Medical education change: a detailed study of six medical schools. Med Educ. 1994;28(5):350–60.

4. Davis MH, Karunathilake I, Harden RM. AMEE Education Guide no. 28: the development and role of departments of medical education. Med Teach. 2005;27(8):665–75.

5. World Federation for Medical Education W. Basic medical education WFME global standards for quality improvement. In: WFME, editor. Copenhagen, Denmark: WFME Office, University of Copenhagen, Denmark; 2003.

6. Grant J, Marshall J, Gary N. Final report: quality improvement in basic medical education evaluation of the implementation in pilot sites of the World Federation for Medical Education's International Standards; 2003.

7. General Medical Council G. Tomorrow's doctors – outcomes and standards for undergraduate medical education. General Medical Council. 2009. Available from: http://www.gmc-uk.org/education/undergraduate/tomorrows_doctors.asp. Cited 20 Feb 2012.

8. General Medical Council G. The trainee doctor – foundation and specialty, including GP training. General Medical Council, GMC. 2011. Available from: http://www.gmc-uk.org/education/postgraduate/standards_and_guidance.asp. Cited 20 Feb 2012.

9. Liaison Committee on Medical Education. Standards for accreditation of medical education programs leading to the M.D. degree Liaison Committee on Medical Education. 2011. Available from: http://www.lcme.org/standard.htm. Cited 20 Feb 2012.

Chapter 2
Mission and Outcomes

All of the accreditation standards in use across the globe articulate the need for the medical education program to define its mission. The statement of the mission is an important way to express the educational philosophy and focus and a means to help the program differentiate itself from other medical education programs. For instance, the mission of a medical school should encapsulate what it is that the medical program wants to achieve now but also define the school's aspirations for the future. Making the medical program mission as succinct as possible such that it is capable of being shared and understood by faculty and students is an important consideration. Most accreditation teams will seek to ensure that the mission is carefully understood by individual members of staff. Mission statements for medical education programs typically describe excellence in teaching (such as innovation) and/or research (such as articulating key research themes or areas). Some medical schools point to course delivery methods such as problem-based or case-based learning and others to the specific context in which student learning will take place (such as rural and remote settings):

> Building on our heritage in surgery, we will enhance human health through endeavour, innovation and collaboration in education, research and service. [1]

G. MacCarrick, *Quality Assurance in Medical Education,*   13
DOI 10.1007/978-0-85729-713-6_2,
© Springer-Verlag London 2013

> As one of the Asia Pacific region's most highly rated education and research institutions, Sydney Medical Program offers unparalleled opportunities to study medicine in Australia... Our graduates play leading roles in health fields around the world and our research investigates diseases which affect millions of lives, including cancer, obesity, chronic disease and ageing, neurosciences and mental health, infectious diseases, and reproductive, maternal and child health. [2]

In some jurisdictions, the program's educational mission addresses indigenous peoples and their health. In all cases, the mission should be defined in consultation with a range of stakeholders such as academic staff and students, the university in which the medical education program sits, the medical profession, health service providers, postgraduate medical training bodies, consumer group representative, and the community.

In addition to the mission, the program must define the outcomes of the program and make these known to stakeholders. The WFME "basic" standard would be deemed to have been met if the medical education program has a clearly defined description of the outcomes and the educational process, leading to a competent doctor fit to practice at a basic level, that is, internship. The WFME "quality" standard would be deemed to have been met if the institutional objectives addressed specific aspects such as social responsibility, research skills, and community engagement and if these have been defined in consultation with relevant stakeholders. In accrediting medical schools in Australia, the Australian Medical Council (AMC) stipulates the need for the school to relate the defined graduate outcomes to the school's mission and to the AMC's goal for medical education, that is, to develop junior doctors who possess attributes that will ensure that they are competent to practice safely and effectively under supervision as interns in Australia or New Zealand. The AMC goes further to point out that the combination of knowledge, skills, and attitudes considered essential for further prevocational and vocational training for medical doctors is very complex and that these attributes cannot be defined simply as lists of factual knowledge, practical skills, or competencies. Equally important attributes of the medical graduate include understanding, problem solving, and appropriate attitudes relevant to caring for individuals who are suffering [3].

The LCME expects senior academic leaders to be familiar with these stated objectives going further to state that the objectives must be stated in "outcome-based terms" that allow assessment of student progress. Outcome-based education has influenced many modern-day medical curricula as a means of making explicit to students what specific knowledge, attitudes, and skills they will acquire by the end of training and by the end of each unit of study [4]. Using an "outcomes-focused" approach ensures that the learning journey is signposted for students and staff. Students can more readily make links between the desired knowledge skills and attitudes and the teaching, learning, and assessment strategies used. The term used is "constructive alignment [4–7]." Accreditation teams will often seek evidence of this alignment between the stated mission and objectives and course delivery and assessment:

> In aligned teaching, there is maximum consistency throughout the system. The curriculum is stated in the form of clear objectives, which state the level of understanding required rather than simply a list of topics to be covered. The teaching methods are chosen that are likely to realise these objectives…the assessment tasks address the objectives… students are "entrapped" in this web of consistency. ([6], p. 27)

In defining curriculum outcomes (as with the school's mission), it is important that these are derived in consultation with relevant stakeholders [8] and that they are cognizant of the various health-care settings in which the school's graduates will work. These outcomes help define the end point of the learning process which is a critical part of the quality improvement process. Some medical schools use the exercise of regularly reviewing curriculum outcomes at annual faculty retreats to ensure the program remains consistent with the school's mission and up to date with advances in health-care practice. Regular review will identify the presence of necessary linkage between outcomes and assessment and help identify possible duplication of teaching effort. There are many published international competency frameworks to inform this process, for example, CanMEDS [9], "Tomorrows Doctors" [10], and the Tuning Project [11],[1] upon which to base a review of the completeness of the stated outcomes of a medical school's curriculum. Many schools group the listed educational outcomes or the "profile" of the ideal medical graduate under "themes" or "domains" which provide a framework to organize the content and delivery of the curriculum as well as student assessment. The use of *themes* to group related curriculum objectives is often used as a means to encourage an important shift away from a traditional discipline-based program to a more integrated approach to medical education. Key champions can be selected from faculty to advocate for particular themes across all years of the program and ensure balance is maintained across the entire curriculum. In addition, the weighting of assessment across themes can be similarly monitored by theme champions. For example, the themes of the undergraduate medical program at the Royal College of Surgeons in Ireland are shown diagrammatically as five interwoven and intersecting strands in Fig. 2.1.

The use of themes provides a framework for the entire program including assessment. Students and trainees typically must demonstrate satisfactory performance in all theme areas in order to graduate.

Once formulated, educational outcomes can be circulated for comment to principal stakeholders. The feedback process should ideally include current students through class representatives, faculty, alumni including recent graduates, patient advocacy groups, and employers of medical graduates. Quality

---

[1]The Tuning Project is the most recent higher education sector-wide initiative to develop learning outcomes/competences for degree qualifications in Europe. Specifically linked to the qualifications framework of the Bologna process, through the MEDINE Thematic Network, a task force led by the University of Edinburgh has developed a framework of learning outcomes for primary medical degree qualifications in Europe (see Cumming and Ross [11]).

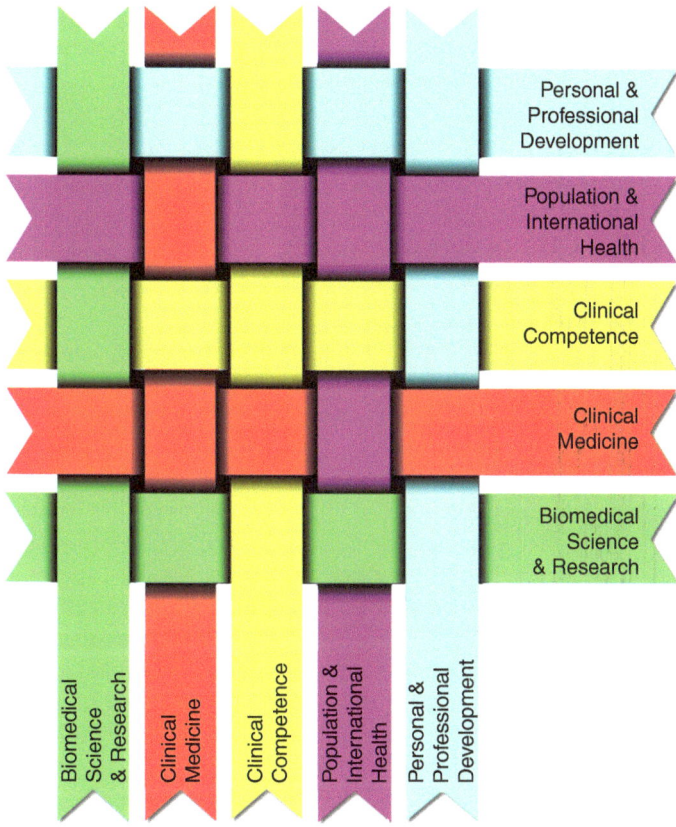

FIGURE 2.1 The five themes of the Medical Program of the Royal College of Surgeons in Ireland

assurance teams are particularly keen to see tangible evidence of a comprehensive consultation process as it attests to the extent to which the program values and is prepared to respond to stakeholder input and concerns. Opportunities for meetings with external stakeholders to discuss the school's missions and outcomes should therefore be carefully recorded and documented. Valuable feedback is often obtained through careful stakeholder consultation, which can assist the program not only in maintaining program outcomes which are current but also in establishing or strengthening important relationships with stakeholders. Recent graduates and alumni are also a rich source of valuable feedback about the adequacy of the stated curriculum outcomes in preparing graduates for internship and beyond.

Documenting Outcomes

As part of the quality assurance process, the program will likely be asked to present examples of learning outcomes. Outcomes are explicit statements of what we want our students and trainees to know, to understand, or to be able to do as a result of completing our courses/training. It is important that faculty understands how to record this information accurately. Learning outcomes are not simply a "wish list" of what we would like students to be capable of doing on completion of the learning activity; rather, they must also be capable of being validly assessed. Accrediting teams will specifically seek evidence of linkage between stated learning outcomes and assessment. Bloom's taxonomy [12] is a very useful aid to writing learning outcomes. The taxonomy consists of a hierarchy of increasingly complex processes which we want our students to acquire. It is vital that learning outcomes are clearly written so that they are understood by students, staff, clinical teachers, and external examiners. When writing learning outcomes, it is helpful to focus on what we expect students to be able to demonstrate upon completion of the module or program. There are several useful resources available on how to write learning outcomes for the medical education setting [13].

Curriculum Database

Finally, an analysis of a medical curriculum beginning with a review of the school's mission and objectives is ideally supported by a curriculum database. Electronic curriculum databases, such as the one shown from the medical school of the University of Melbourne (reproduced with permission), are typically organized by theme and also searchable by topics and keywords (see Figs. 2.2 and 2.3). Documenting the curriculum in such a format will assist curriculum planners, faculty, and students.

Such a tool, if available, is often requested by accreditation teams to determine the extent to which material has been covered in the curriculum as well as the depth, breadth, and integration of specific themes or domains. CurrMIT© is one such a tool widely used in the United States of America and Canada which uses a relational database containing curriculum information such as outcomes, resources, content, educational methods, assessment methods, and educational sites. The University of New South Wales, Faculty of Medicine in Australia, has also developed its own curriculum management system called eMed©. This system not only manages graduate outcomes, content, and activities but also the results of program evaluation.

As most medical programs operate a distributed model of medical education, it is critical that all teaching sites are familiar with the learning outcomes, not only for their particular component of the program but also for that which is to follow. A well-designed curriculum management tool can assist by providing easy access to those parts of the curriculum that need to be viewed and managed centrally as well as those that need to be viewed and managed by staff and students at multiple sites. A key aspect of the curriculum database for quality assurance is that it demonstrates linkage between learning outcomes, assessment, and evaluation. The example Fig. 2.4 represented on a simple excel spread sheet links unit or module learning outcomes to the weekly learning objectives and to the relevant overarching theme/domain, as well as to the proposed assessment format.

MD CURRICULUM DATABASE
LOGGED IN: **STAFF** (LOGOUT)

Search database   Search

Change Year (Current view: **Year 2012**)   Year 2 Forms and Clinical Skills Communication Modules

YEAR	BLOCK	WEEK	ACTIVITY
Year 1 ▲	Foundation	4. Atherosclerosis	Lecture 1. Drugs influencing heart rate and arrhythmias
Year 2	**Cardiovascular** ▲	5. AMI	Lecture 2. Superior and posterior mediastinum
Year 3	Respiratory	**6. Complete heart block** ▲	Lecture 3. Aetiology and risk factors for CVD
Year 4	Gastrointestinal	7. Valve problems	Lecture 4. Observational studies in CVD
	Renal		Lecture 5. Lungs and pleura
	Revision		Lecture 6. Introduction to pharmacokinetics
	Student conference		Lecture 7. Antibiotics 1: Classification, targets of action
	Neurosciences		Lecture 8. Antibiotics 2: Development and basis of resistance
	Endocrine		Lecture 9. Ischemic heart disease
	Metabolism		Lecture 10. Antibiotics 3: Choosing and using antibiotics
	Locomotor		Practical. Bacteraemia and septicaemia
	Exercise		PCP1 tutorial. Tutorial 6
	Reproduction		Clinical colloquium. Clinical colloquium
	Intersystem integration		Tutorial. Challenges for public health
	Skin		CSL tutorial (session 1). Eleanor fogarty
			CSL tutorial (session 2). Eleanor fogarty
			Practical. Blood pressure, genes and sodium (post-treatment data) (Week 5)

© COPYRIGHT 2012 **MELBOURNE MEDICAL SCHOOL** | **TECHNICAL SUPPORT**

FIGURE 2.2 Example of searchable curriculum database showing learning activities by week, block, and year (Reproduced with permission from University of Melbourne)

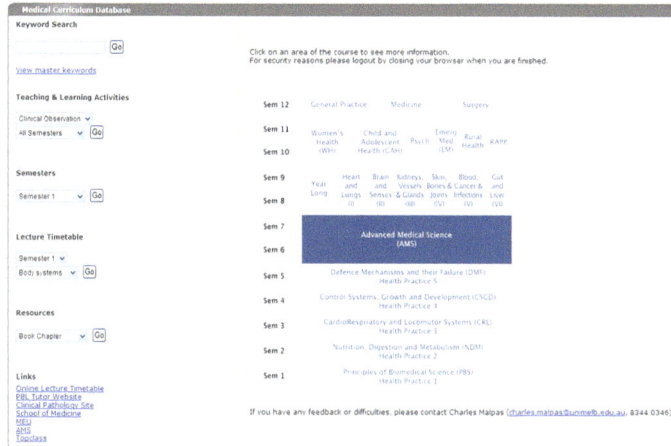

FIGURE 2.3 Most databases include a keyword search function, mapping all teaching and learning activities in the curriculum to specific learning outcomes

Unit Learning Outcome No.	Unit Learning Outcome	Theme No.	Weekly Learning Objective Nos.	Sub Outcome No. (MGP No.)	Suggested Assessment
U101.11	Describe the structure and function of a cell.	1	101.2.11; 101.3.13; 101.3.14	S1.1, S1.2	MCQs; EMQs; SAQs
			101.3.15; 101.3.16; 101.4.13		
			101.4.14; 101.5.12; 101.5.14		
			101.5.15; 101.5.16; 101.7.13		
			101.8.15; 101.9.13; 101.9.14		
			101.9.15; 101.10.14; 101.11.11		
			101.11.12; 101.11.13; 101.11.14		
			101.12.15		
U101.12	Describe the structure and explain the function of the tissue types.	1	101.1.11; 101.1.12; 101.1.16	S1.1, S1.2	MCQs; EMQs; SAQs
			101.1.17; 101.1.18; 101.1.19		WebCT
			101.2.18; 101.3.16; 101.5.11		
			101.6.13; 101.6.14; 101.7.11		
			101.7.12; 101.8.13; 101.8.14		
			101.8.16; 101.8.17; 101.9.11		
			101.9.12; 101.9.14; 101.9.15		
			101.10.11; 101.10.12; 101.10.13		
			101.10.14; 101.10.15; 101.11.14		
			101.11.15		
U101.13	Describe the structure and explain the function of the skin and its derivatives.	1	101.2.12; 101.2.17; 101.3.11	S1.1, S1.2; S1.3	MCQs; EMQs; SAQs
			101.3.12; 101.4.11; 101.4.12		iPEs
			101.5.13; 101.7.12; 101.7.14		
			101.10.16; 101.12.12		
U101.14	Explain the principles of inflammation, tissue injury and repair.	1	101.2.17; 101.3.17; 101.4.12	S1.3	MCQs; EMQs; SAQs
			101.4.15; 101.6.15; 101.8.16		
			101.8.110; 101.9.18; 101.10.16		
			101.11.16; 101.11.17; 101.12.11		
			101.12.12; 101.12.15		
U101.15	Describe the structure and function of biomolecules associated with the life process.	1	101.2.13; 101.2.14; 101.2.14	S1.1; S2.1	MCQs; EMQs; SAQs
			101.2.16; 101.3.16; 101.5.15		
			101.8.18; 101.8.19; 101.8.111		
			101.9.16		
U101.16	Explain the physiological principles of homeostasis.	1	101.1.13; 101.1.14; 101.1.15	S1.1; S2.1	MCQs; EMQs; SAQs
			101.6.11; 101.6.11; 101.6.12		
			101.7.14; 101.9.16; 101.9.17		
U101.17	Describe at an introductory level the basic principles of microbiology.	1	101.5.16; 101.11.18; 101.12.13	S2.1	MCQs; EMQs; SAQs
			101.12.14		
U101.18	Apply basic First-Aid principles in a simulated environment.	1	101.2.31; 101.6.15; 101.7.31	S4.2; S5.1; S6.1	MCQs; EMQs; SAQs
			101.8.110		
U101.21	Describe principles of interpersonal communication and apply generic communication skills.	2	101.2.21; 101.2.23; 101.3.25	S8.1	EMQs; WebCT
			101.4.21; 101.5.21; 101.6.21		
			101.7.21; 101.8.21; 101.9.21		
			101.10.21; 101.11.21; 101.12.21		
U101.22	Discuss the importance of communication in medical practice.	2	101.5.21; 101.6.21; 101.7.21	S8.1	EMQs; WebCT; TR
			101.8.21; 101.11.21; 101.12.21		
U101.23	Describe the theoretical principles that underpin collaborative teamwork.	2	101.2.24; 101.2.32; 101.2.41	S9.1	EMQs; WebCT
			101.3.21; 101.3.22; 101.3.23		
			101.4.41; 101.7.31; 101.11.21		
			101.12.21		

FIGURE 2.4 A simple excel spread can be used to demonstrate linkage between overarching theme learning outcomes, unit learning outcomes, and weekly learning objectives as well as to the planned assessment strategies

Summary Points

- Statements of the medical program mission are an important way to express a medical schools' educational philosophy and focus and a means to help the program differentiate itself from other programs.
- Defining the end point of the learning process is a critical first step in the quality improvement process. The medical school's mission and objectives will inform all subsequent aspects of the quality assurance process.
- The medical program objectives should be developed in close consultation with all stakeholders and need to be cognizant of the various health-care settings in which the medical graduates will work.
- There are several published international competency frameworks, which can inform the process of defining curriculum outcomes.
- A careful examination of the school's curriculum using a searchable database can yield important information about the necessary linkages between stated objectives, delivery methods, and assessment as well as help to identify possible duplication of teaching effort.

References

1. Royal College of Surgeons in Ireland R. Noble purpose. Dublin: Royal College of Surgeons in Ireland; 2012. Available from: http://www.rcsi.ie/. Cited 20 Feb 2012.
2. Sydney Medical School. The University of Sydney. 2012. Available from: http://sydney.edu.au/medicine/. Cited 20 Feb 2012.
3. Australian Medical Council Limited. Standards for assessment and accreditation of medical schools by the Australian Medical Council 2010. Australian Medical Council Limited; 2010.
4. Harden RM. Outcome-based education: the future is today. Med Teach. 2007;29(7):625–9.

5. Harden RM. Outcome-based education – the ostrich, the peacock and the beaver. Med Teach. 2007;29(7):666–71.
6. Biggs J. Teaching for quality learning at university. 2nd ed. Buckingham: Open University Press; 2003.
7. Harden RM. Learning outcomes as a tool to assess progression. Med Teach. 2007;29(7):678–82.
8. Kassebaum DG, Eaglen RH, Cutler ER. The objectives of medical education: reflections in the accreditation looking glass. Acad Med. 1997;72(7):648–56.
9. Frank JR, Danoff D. The CanMEDS initiative: implementing an outcomes-based framework of physician competencies. Med Teach. 2007;29(7):642–7.
10. General Medical Council G. Tomorrows doctors. 2008. Available from: http://www.gmc-uk.org/education/undergraduate/undergraduate_policy/tomorrows_doctors.asp#Introduction. Cited Dec 2008.
11. Cumming A, Ross M. The Tuning Project for Medicine – learning outcomes for undergraduate medical education in Europe. Med Teach. 2007;29(7):636–41.
12. Bloom B, Englehart M, Furst E, Hill W, Krathwohl D. Taxonomy of educational objectives: the classification of educational goals. New York/Toronto: Longmans, Green; 1956.
13. Kennedy D. Writing and using learning outcomes: a practical guide. Ireland: University College Cork; 2007.

Chapter 3
The Educational Program

This chapter examines the educational program offered by a medical institution, the adequacy of the content of the program, the instructional methods used to deliver the program, how the program is managed, and how the program is linked with other stages of the medical education continuum.

Apart from a description of the curriculum's overarching objectives, most accrediting teams will seek evidence of a preplanned curriculum model and confirmation that a range of instructional methods are used to deliver the program. It should be possible for a visiting team to view the curriculum at a glance. Figure 3.1 provides an overview of the entire program which can then be further examined module by module. In the case of undergraduate medical education programs, the description of the program should make clear where the exit points are located, that is, where students can exit the medical program and receive credit for mastered learning. The placement of electives and research opportunities should also be made clear to a visiting team. Some jurisdictions require evidence of a minimum period of instruction; for instance, the LCME requires evidence of 130 weeks. The AMC stipulates that a typical requirement of a minimum course length of five calendar years for an undergraduate-entry course and 4 years for a graduate-entry course. The depth of coverage of the

G. MacCarrick, *Quality Assurance in Medical Education,*
DOI 10.1007/978-0-85729-713-6_3,
© Springer-Verlag London 2013

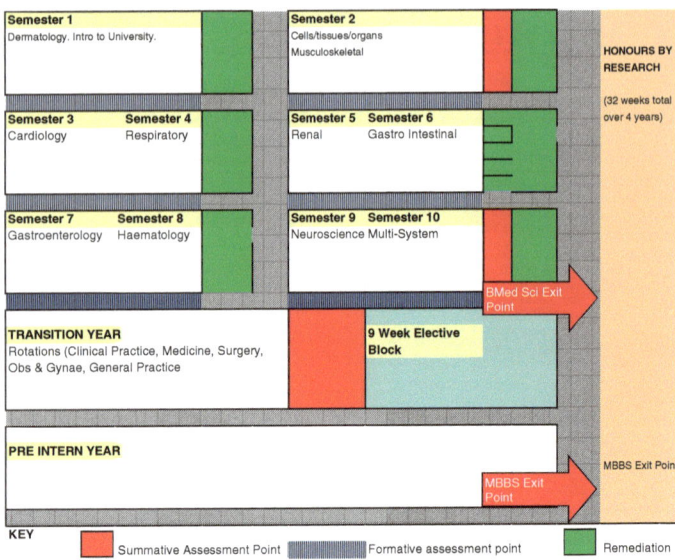

FIGURE 3.1 The overview of the medical program should indicate the timing of remediation (if required), electives, and opportunities to engage in research. Likewise, it should be clear where students can exit the medical program and receive credit for mastered learning

individual topics will depend on the medical education program's educational goals and objectives.

Examples of week-by-week instruction are also a useful submission to include in documentation to an accrediting team. If the educational program mission purports to use a particular educational approach, for example, problem-based learning [1], then this should be evident in the weekly learning. Figure 3.2 is an example week arranged around a clinical case. Each of the teaching strategies employed helps deliver the outcomes associated with the clinical case. Students meet at the start of each week to discuss the clinical case, meet again in tutorial sessions midweek to answer questions (a clinician and member of academic staff are present), and again at the end of the week to present back to the larger group on key tasks that were

	Monday	Tuesday	Wednesday	Thursday	Friday
0900 – 1000	Lecture 1: Case Introduced: Spinal Cord Injury	Lecture 4: Nervous System 5: Development of the nervous system	Lecture 6: (Biomed Staff) Nervous System 7: The synapse and spinal cord reflexes	Practical 1 (3-week rotation) Communication and Collaboration (Clinician)	Practical 4 (3-week rotation) (Integrated Exploration) Nervous System Upper Limb
1000 – 1100	Small Group A (Facilitated) Case Outline and Task Allocation		Tutorial 1: (Clinician and MS Staff) Review of case development	Principles of eliciting a family and social history	Vertebral Column
1100 – 1200	Small Group B (Facilitated) Case Outline and Task Allocation		Tutorial 2: (Clinician and Biomed Staff) Review of case development	Practical 2 (3-week rotation) (Clinician) Clinical Examination of	Small Group A (Facilitated)
1200 – 1300	Lecture 2: (Rehab Specialist) Long-term management of the spinal cord injured patient	Lecture 5: (Biomed Staff) Nervous System 6 The spinal cord		the Lower Limb	Small Group B
Lunch					
1400 – 1500	Lecture 3: (Biomed Staff) Overview of the upper limb.	Information Literacy Development:(Library staff) End Note – Review of Skills	Community visit (Theme 3)	Lecture 7: Intro to Neuromuscular Pathology	Case Wrap-up & student task presentations:
1500 – 1600				Practical 3 (3-week rotation) (Dissection)	
1600 – 1700				Dissection of the lower limb continuing…	
Extra curricular			Asynchronous on-line discussion	Web-based formative assessment	

FIGURE 3.2 Example of instruction based around a weekly clinical case

assigned. In addition, timetabled practical sessions complement the learning with dissection, explorations, and workshops on communication and clinical skills.

The particular type of educational strategies the school embraces will depend on resources available. The school should be aware of the shortcomings of whatever strategy is used. If cases or problems are being used, then it is expected that faculty will understand how this method helps address key learning objectives. It is particularly important that both clinical and nonclinical staff are familiar with the clinical case each week so that links can be made to assist student learning.

A commonly used curriculum method used by medical schools to help consolidate student learning over time is the spiral curriculum [2–4]. The notion that underpins the spiral curriculum is that key learning objectives are revisited regularly throughout the course, thereby reinforcing learning. The use of a virtual learning environment, which enables students to create and record their progress and experience over time, supports such a model by encouraging students to revisit material taught earlier in the program. This is particularly important in the postgraduate setting where trainees are encouraged to link theory, much of which is acquired in basic medical education, to practice.

When representing the curriculum to an external review team, it can be useful to represent the curriculum's strengths on a continuum using, for example, the SPICES model. Harden [5] identified six key educational strategies that relate to the curriculum in any medical school. Each issue can be represented as a spectrum or continuum: student centered/teacher centered, problem based/information gathering, integrated discipline based, community based/hospital based, elective/uniform, and systematic/apprenticeship based. A useful exercise prior to a site visit is for faculty to consider where the program "sits" on this continuum and where it would like to be in the future. A program which is in transition may choose to capture its current versus proposed model as follows:

Student centered	↓		↓			Teacher centered
Problem based		↓			↓	Information gathering
Integrated	↓				↓	Discipline
Community		↓			↓	Hospital
Elective			↓	↓		Uniform
Systematic		↓↓				Apprentice
Key:	↓ = Profile of the current program			↓ = Proposed profile		

The blue arrows suggest a more traditional curriculum, which relies on traditional educational approaches. The red arrow indicates the proposed program, i.e. where the school aims to be in the future in terms of SPICES model. By examining each of the components of Harden's SPICES model, staff can gain a better understanding of the direction in which they wish to take the medical program into the future. As part of the quality assurance process, faculty *and* students should examine the extent to which the program is perceived as student centered. Questions which might be asked of the program by a quality assurance team would include: Are students/trainees actively encouraged to take more responsibility for their own learning? Is the emphasis on the students and on what and how they learn? (in contrast to a teacher-centered approach, where the emphasis is on the teachers and what they teach). The support provided for student/trainee learning will be carefully examined by a visiting team. Such support can begin prior to new students commencing the program with face-to-face lectures and tutorials or online tutorials covering aspects such as how to access and effectively utilize the medical school's learning resources and understanding the process of preparing for assessment. Recent graduates about to commence internship can likewise be provided online orientation prior to commencement of their supervised training. The model and instructional strategies employed should ensure that students are encouraged to incrementally take responsibility for their own learning, becoming more self-directed as the course progresses. In the postgraduate sector in particular, training should focus on ensuring increasing independence as learners as skills, knowledge, and experience increase.

The emphasis of many traditional programs has been to provide students with a large body of basic science and clinical knowledge. Once qualified, students are expected to be able to synthesize this information and apply it to the care of their patients. The reality is that this approach does not adequately prepare students for their careers as doctors. In medical education, the delivery of course objectives can potentially utilize a wide variety of modes of delivery including the traditional lecture, case-based learning (where a clinical case is used to illustrate or contextualize learning), small group tutorials (both staff and student directed), practicals (e.g., anatomy dissection), computer-assisted learning, bedside clinical teaching; grand rounds, shadowing, skills workshops, sitting in with consultants, theatre attendance, ward attendance, and home visits. There are advantages and disadvantages to each educational method. It is important that the educational method chosen supports the curriculum objectives and is feasible. To accommodate the many different learner styles, it is important that no one instructional strategy predominates.

For instance, an overemphasis on didactic lectures will not achieve a medical school's mission of producing graduates skilled and committed to self-directed learning. Of all the three domains of learning (cognitive, psychomotor, and affective), the cognitive domain is clearly important in medical education as recall and recognition of specific facts, procedures, patterns, and concepts are important aspects of the intellectual development of the medical graduate. However, it is equally important that the other two domains of learning, the affective domain (which includes motivation and attitudes) and the psychomotor domain (which includes motor-skill areas requiring practice and precision), are also embraced as part of the curriculum. An accrediting team will look for evidence of use of a *variety* of teaching and learning strategies and that the educational strategies chosen maintain congruence with the stated objectives of the curriculum.

In the traditional basic medical education curriculum, teaching in the early years tended to emphasize the classical disciplines such as anatomy, physiology, biochemistry, and pathology. Contact with patients tended to occur after completion of the basic science component of the medical curriculum. This preclinical to clinical sequence is increasingly being challenged by the need to contextualize theoretical learning and to facilitate professional socialization from an earlier point in the curriculum. Quality assurance teams will specifically seek evidence of initiatives that aim to enhance the clinical relevance of teaching in the biomedical sciences and evidence of revisiting concepts from the biomedical sciences in the clinical years. There should be adequate opportunity for both horizontal (within a course section) and vertical (across successive course sections) integration of subject material. The latter should provide opportunities for students to revisit course material covered earlier in the course.

The context for learning is another important consideration. Changing case mix in hospitals, with shorter lengths of stay, means that hospitals may not be the ideal teaching ground they once were. Increasingly, the ambulatory care and community setting is being utilized as legitimate training environments for both basic and postgraduate medical education.

Elective programs in a curriculum give students the opportunity to select subjects or projects of their own choosing (often in a different health-care setting) and are an important aspect of any medical program. Elective study also creates space within the curriculum for stronger students to compete for higher honors and for weaker students to achieve the core. The elective program also provides opportunities for students to pursue research activity.

Curriculum Content

Most quality assurance teams will request details about the content of the curriculum. All international standards require the principles of scientific method, and evidence-based medicine must be embedded throughout the curriculum. Students must be capable of using scientific principles and skills of problem solving. Graduates should have sufficient understanding of the scientific underpinnings of medicine such that these can be applied in the clinical setting. A particular aspect which most accrediting teams will explore is the extent to which the biomedical science content is clinically relevant. It is important that input from clinicians is sought in both the planning and delivery of the biomedical sciences teaching particularly in the early years where the biomedical sciences traditionally predominate. Likewise, it is important that biomedical scientists participate in the planning and delivery of intermediate and later years of the program where typically bedside clinical teaching predominates.

The curriculum should inculcate analytical and critical thinking and include specific laboratory, hands-on, or simulated (e.g., computer based) exercises in which students collect, analyze, and interpret data and test hypotheses. The ethical principles underpinning clinical and translational research should also be addressed in the curriculum including how research is conducted, how studies are evaluated, and patient consent and explanation.

Most medical schools have a strong research focus, thereby providing adequate opportunity to make research awareness, understanding, and evaluation a strong component of the curriculum. The challenge however is to ensure that all students graduate competent in research skills not just those who self-select research electives or placements. An additional challenge can be ensuring a balance between opportunities for research experience in not only the biomedical sciences but also the social and behavioral sciences. In the postgraduate setting, the focus on research should build on the basic medical education with trainees continuing to acquire skills in critical appraisal of the literature, evidence-based medicine and research methodology.

The behavioral and social sciences and medical ethics should be adequately addressed in both basic and postgraduate medical programs. Included in this are important aspects of professionalism such as the ability to work collaboratively with colleagues; recognizing one's own strengths and weaknesses; understanding the legal and ethical responsibilities of a medical practitioner; and commitment to lifelong learning, self-appraisal, and reflection. The complexities and dilemmas of clinical practice should also be explored in terms of different cultural and religious backgrounds.

Increasingly, the planned use of portfolios (see Fig. 3.3) enables students and trainees to maintain a log of self and peer reviews, supervisor reports, reflective journals, certification in professional skills such as script writing, and informed consent. The use of portfolios in the postgraduate setting can also include recording of trainee's experience of critical incidents as well as recording emerging strengths and weaknesses as trainees progress through the program.

A growing challenge for most medical schools and postgraduate training programs is ensuring adequacy of clinical contact and time for structured reflection on clinical experience. A number of factors frustrate efforts to guarantee sufficient clinical experience including shorter patient lengths of stay in hospitals. Accrediting teams will often examine clinical rotations carefully to ensure schools protect sufficient

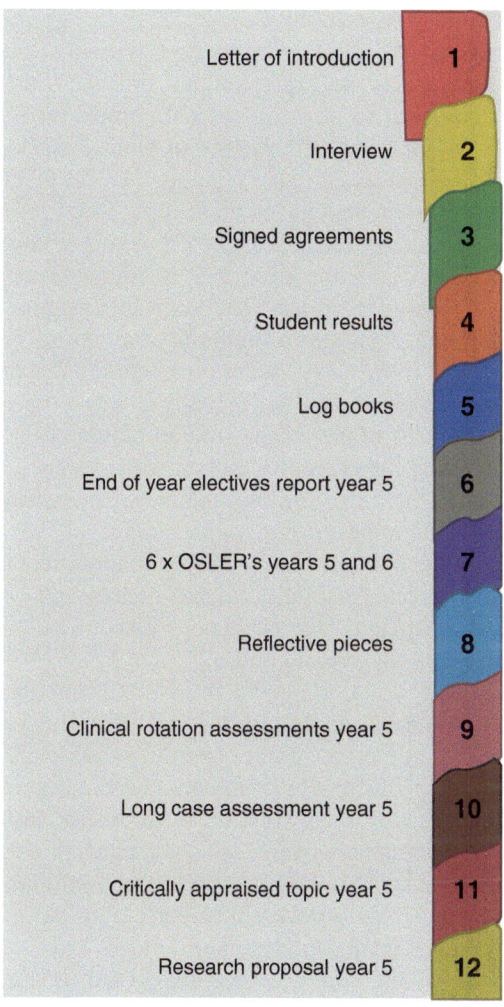

FIGURE 3.3 Example table of contents of a student portfolio

time for formal clinical teaching in their affiliated hospitals. A significant period of time should be devoted to students' direct contact with patients. The AMC recommends a period equivalent to at least 2 years spent primarily in direct contact with patients, as well as contact with patients during other parts of the course, and recommends that the most effective way for students to develop clinical competence and judgment is participation in a variety of clinical clerkships. The use of skills centers can also enhance clinical teaching, providing a safe environment for students to practice procedures and skills including team-based skills. Another challenge for most medical education programs is adequate exposure to community-based practice. Residents in long-stay facilities are often used to augment community-based or general practice rotations. In this way, students can commence their exposure to the "real" clinical setting earlier in the program.

In the context of increasing student numbers, the program should provide the accrediting team with evidence of targets for staff/student ratios and any plans for increasing clinical placements. The latter is typically achieved through the phased expansion of affiliated clinical schools, increasing utilization of private hospitals, nursing homes, and community health organizations for systematic placement of students and trainees in the private and other public sectors.

Where a distributed model is in place, the school must ensure educational experiences at all sites are designed to achieve the same educational objectives. Although the types and frequency of clinical problems and conditions seen at each site may vary, each rotation must ensure that students receive sufficient exposure to core clinical experiences. Similarly, time spent in hospital, community, and other ambulatory settings must ensure equivalence and that any limitations in site learning environments need to be addressed. Students must encounter curriculum content related to each phase of the human life cycle and be capable of recognizing and interpreting symptoms and signs of disease in all organ systems. Traditional disciplines such as family medicine/general practice, internal medicine, obstetrics and gynecology, pediatrics, preventive medicine, psychiatry, and surgery should all be represented in the curriculum. It is also expected that the curriculum examines the interface between orthodox and complementary practices. Modern health practitioners need to be aware that some patients will choose to use a range of alternative therapies and that some of these will not be supported by evidence. Graduates must be aware of these and how they might affect other proposed treatment plans.

Basic and postgraduate medical education programs should ensure adequate instruction in communication skills including communication with patients and their families, colleagues, and other health professionals as well as patients from different cultural backgrounds. Specific instruction should also be provided in medical ethics and human values before students engage in direct patient contact. As students take on increasingly more active roles in patient care, there should be a means for identifying possible breaches of ethics in patient care. The LCME uses the term "scrupulous ethical principles" to include characteristics such as honesty, integrity, maintenance of confidentiality, and respect for patients, patients' families, other students, and other health professionals. Studies in communication, ethics, law, psychology, sociology, and other behavioral and social sciences would be regarded as providing grounding in the principles of professionalism and ethical decision making.

In 2005, the General Medical Council (GMC) and the Medical Schools Council (MSC) established the joint *Student Fitness to Practise Working Group* which developed guidance for medical schools and their students relating to the professional behavior expected of medical students. This guidance recognizes that medical students have unique responsibilities, and as such different standards of professional behavior are required [6].

Additional aspects a visiting team will examine include curriculum content relating to quality assurance in health care, including systems management. Students need to understand how errors can happen in practice and the principles of managing risk. An extension of this is the recognition that health-care delivery can be greatly enhanced by the coordinated contributions of professionals from different backgrounds working together as a team. Students should be exposed to the roles and functions of different health-care providers with dedicated instruction on interprofessional education. At a postgraduate level, the training content would be expected to extend beyond this to include public health policy, medical jurisprudence, and health-care management.

Management of the Program

As part of the quality assurance process, each medical education program must demonstrate that its program is appropriately governed. In the medical school, typically a central curriculum committee operates which includes on its membership staff students and external stakeholders. Such a committee should have sufficient authority to plan, implement, and regularly revise the curriculum. Such a committee should also have at its disposal sufficient resources to support innovation. Accrediting teams will often examine carefully the resource allocation model in place in the school and seek input from faculty and students as to the extent to which consultation takes place in designing, implementing, and resourcing the curriculum. The management of postgraduate training (example shown below) must likewise clearly identify what structures are in place for organizing, delivering, resourcing, coordinating, managing, and assessing the training process. The responsible body should have adequate representation from trainees and teaching staff. Training should be regarded as complementary and not subordinate to the service requirements of training posts.

The quality assurance process will require the medical education program to demonstrate sufficient liaison and links with prior or subsequent stages of medical training. For example, medical schools will need to demonstrate an awareness of the needs of the different health service environments in which its graduates will be working. The school's alumni office is often a useful resource in this regard and can assist by collating graduate tracking data and administrating graduate surveys. Links with postgraduate training bodies will ensure that the curriculum remains current and responsive. Likewise, the structure and composition of postgraduate training programs should be able to demonstrate the relationship with both basic medical education and subsequent health-care delivery.

Summary Points

- A range of instructional methods should be used to deliver the program which utilizes all three domains of learning (cognitive, psychomotor, and affective).
- There should be adequate opportunity for both horizontal and vertical integration of subject material.
- There should be a strong nexus demonstrated between the program's research and teaching.
- Adequacy of clinical contact in a variety of health-care settings is an important consideration.
- The program resource allocation model should be transparent.
- Program management should be representative of key stakeholders.

References

1. Barrows HS. A taxonomy of problem-based learning methods. Med Educ. 1986;20(6):481–6.
2. Bruner JS. The process of education. New York: Vintage Books; 1960.
3. Masters K, Gibbs T. The spiral curriculum: implications for online learning. BMC Med Educ. 2007;7:52.
4. Harden RM. What is a spiral curriculum? Med Teach. 1999;21(2):141–3.
5. Harden RM, Sowden S, Dunn WR. Educational strategies in curriculum development: the SPICES model. Med Educ. 1984 Jul;18(4):284–97.
6. General Medical Council G. Medical students: professional values and fitness to practise. General Medical Council, GMC. 2005. Available from: http://www.gmc-uk.org/education/undergraduate/professional_behaviour.asp. Cited 20 Feb 2012.

Chapter 4
Assessment of Learning

> No single assessment method can provide all the data required for judgement of anything so complex as the delivery of professional services by a successful physician. [1]

This chapter examines the quality assurance aspects of assessing student learning. The terms assessment and evaluation are sometimes used interchangeably. For the purposes of this book, "assessment" is reserved for the description of activities which measure medical student knowledge, performance, and attitudes, while the term "evaluation" is reserved for faculty, student, course, and clinical rotation appraisal and feedback.

An examination of a medical programs assessment strategy will aim to establish whether the program of assessment is systematic, valid, and reliable. Importantly, the assessment should reflect the educational objectives of the curriculum and be capable of identifying students who are underperforming. The overall program should utilize a variety of assessment formats, and accompanying the assessment strategy, there should be in place robust plans for remediation.

Most schools will have an assessment policy which informs faculty and students about matters relating to assessment. This will typically contain information such as the assessment blueprint [2] which will ensure that each assessment is based on appropriate sampling of the program learning outcomes. The assessment policy should also describe the basis for and timing of formative[1] and summative[2] assessments, rules related to attendance, the different types of knowledge-based and performance-based assessments in use, process for managing poorly performing and fitness to practice issues such as health or personal issues, and professionalism. This guide should also make explicit rules relating to student progression.

The emphasis of the assessment strategy should be on judging student mastery of knowledge, skills, and attitudes, measuring improvement over time, diagnosing student difficulties, and motivating students to learn and to take responsibility for their own ongoing learning and professional development. A focus should be to provide high-quality formative assessment, through regular feedback. The purpose of each component of the assessment should be clearly defined for students and trainees ensuring the content derives from and represents the breadth of the curriculum. The workload associated with assessment needs to be carefully monitored so as not to detract from ongoing learning. The design of the assessment program must be based on fair and timely formative and summative assessment.

In the case of medical schools which typically fall under the auspices of a university, it should be clear how the assessment rules and regulations of the medical school and the parent organization are reconciled. This may be particularly important for the awarding of university prizes, etc. While generic attributes of the university graduate will typically apply to the medical school,[3] most medical schools require additional specific discipline-related attributes required of

---

[1] Formative assessment is intended to modify and to inform student learning. Formative methods of assessment generally precede a summative assessment method and are not part of the official student record of achievement.

[2] Summative assessment evaluates mastery of the learning objectives of the course, forms part or all of the final result, and determines progression within the course.

[3] Most Universities require specific attributes be achieved by all university graduates. Typically these include; Knowledge, Communication skills Problem-solving skills, International perspective and Social responsibility.

the profession. The assessment methods chosen by a medical school must provide a comprehensive assessment of the core knowledge, skills, and attitudes required of a medical graduate. Medical student and trainee assessment should include direct observation of the core clinical skills, behaviors, and attitudes that have been specified in the program's educational objectives. There should be regular assessment of problem solving, clinical reasoning, decision making, and communication skills. Faculty and trainers should understand the purposes and benefits of different types of assessment and the uses and limitations of various test formats, for instance, criterion-referenced versus norm-referenced assessment and formative versus summative assessment. Faculty should have access to individuals who are knowledgeable about the different methods for assessment in medical education, and the institution should provide adequate opportunities for faculty to develop and enhance their skills in such methods.

Assessment Methods Chosen

The medical education program must be able to clearly describe the various methods used to assess acquisition of knowledge skills and attitudes. For example, assessing knowledge may be achieved using multiple choice questions [3], extended matching items [4], key features testing [5], or constructed response questions [6]. Assessing skills may be achieved using OSCEs [7], and measurement of acquisition of appropriate attributes such as professionalism can be explored using portfolios [8]. It is useful for the medical education program to quantify the overall amount of assessment which takes place in any defined period of the program including the breakdown of formative and summative assessment and different assessment formats (see Fig. 4.1).

In addition medical education programs will typically be asked to produce evidence of measures of reliability and validity of assessment methods in use. In addition, evidence will be sought that any new assessment approaches the school

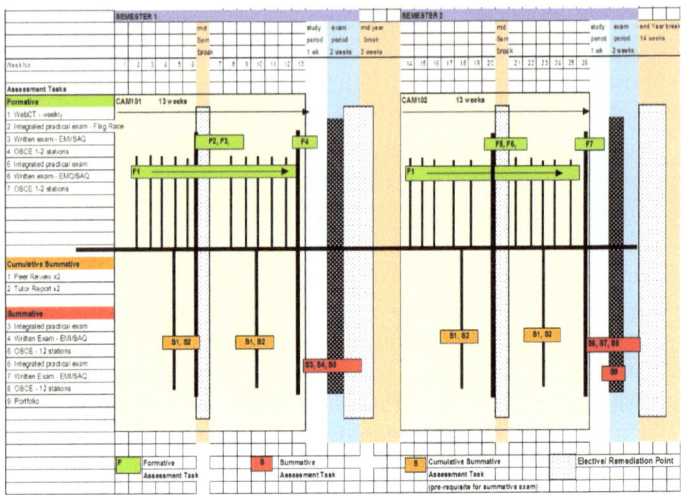

FIGURE 4.1 Assessment plan showing key summative and formative assessment points

has introduced are being evaluated. Van der Vleuten [9] describes five helpful criteria for determining the usefulness of a particular method of assessment: reliability (the degree to which the measurement is accurate and reproducible), validity (whether the assessment measures what it claims to measure), impact on future learning and practice, acceptability to learners and faculty, and the cost of assessment. Evidence of standard setting [10] will be particularly relevant for high-stakes assessments. The medical education program should be able to demonstrate which particular form of standard setting is in use and how the results are used to set the pass mark. Assessment in medical education is the subject of a growing body of research and literature, and as such considerable technical expertise is required. Each program should consider the best way of acquiring this expertise either through consultancy and/or in-house faculty development.

Table 4.1 shows the results of a typical standard setting exercise and the results which might be submitted in evidence of how the pass mark was reached on sample assessment

TABLE 4.1 Example of results obtained using Angoff method

Question	Judge 1	Judge 2	Judge 3	Judge 4	Average
1	0.60	0.65	0.70	0.65	0.65
2	0.40	0.30	0.40	0.50	0.4
3	0.30	0.70	0.50	0.50	0.5
4	0.50	0.40	0.50	0.60	0.5
5	0.65	0.70	0.75	0.70	0.7
					2.75

$$\text{Pass mark} = \frac{2.75}{5} \times 100 \rightarrow 55\%$$

items. Typically, a Medical Education Unit can provide and or coordinate capacity building in the specific areas of assessment including item writing, station construction for OSCEs, and standard setting for both written and clinical examinations.

Authentic clinical examinations, whether using real or simulated patients, should form a significant component of the overall assessment plan. Clinical examinations should include an assessment of student ability to recognize abnormal clinical findings (and their distinction from normal) and the ability to provide an appropriate interpretation of these findings.

The Key Relationship Between Assessment and Learning

Improving integration of various assessment formats to encourage deep learning as well as reducing assessment "overload" is an important consideration. Quality assurance teams are generally keen to ensure that students are not over-assessed. Overemphasis on summative assessment in particular generally detracts from the capacity of students to extend their learning beyond the taught curriculum. It is important to review the quantum and timing of assessment to ensure that the assessments from one area of the program do not impact on the teaching and learning activities from other parts of the program. Present-day approaches to assessment in medical education emphasize a systematic and programmatic approach based on multiple aggregated measures of the student's knowledge, skill, and abilities over time [11]. There should be a feasible assessment plan with a workload requirement that can be reasonably met by students. The assessment schedule should be fully disclosed in a timely fashion to enable students to allocate sufficient time to meet all other commitments. Figure 4.1, for example, provides information about the planned timing of each assessment including where and how students can expect to receive feedback. Where students are required to undertake additional or supplementary examinations, it is appropriate that opportunities for remediation are made available. Sometimes, it is recognized that this is not always possible under some university examination rules.

As with instructional methods chosen, assessment should focus on all three domains of learning (cognitive, psychomotor, and affective). Accrediting teams will be particularly keen to see evidence of assessment strategies which explore the professional domains of practice such as interpersonal skills, accountability, and ethics. Also, as part of the quality assurance process, the medical education program will be evaluated on its attempts to ensure consistency in approached to assessment across all clinical teaching sites. It is vital that all faculty involved with teaching are adequately briefed on the assessment requirements. In addition, faculty who have direct responsibility for the assessment of medical student or trainee performance should understand the uses and limitations of the various assessment formats, reliability and validity issues, formative versus summative assessment, and other factors associated with effective educational assessment.

Any plans to use a virtual learning environment to deliver assessments on line (e.g., project work, MCQs, and uploading of electronic portfolios) will be carefully examined by a

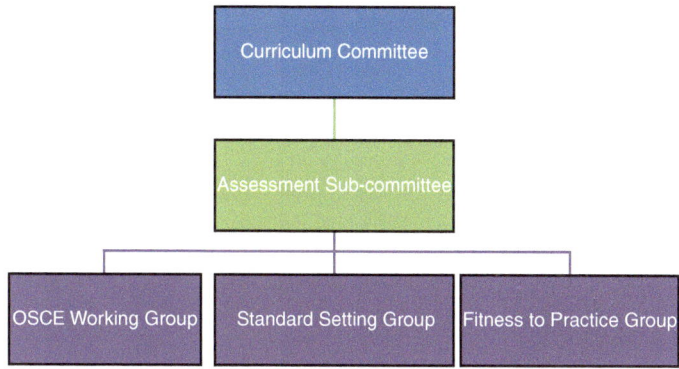

FIGURE 4.2 The assessment committee typically has several working groups responsible for reviewing assessment procedures and guidelines such as fitness to practice, standard setting, and OSCEs

quality assurance team to ensure it is used with care and sensitivity, if it is to add value to the overall learning experience.

Typically, the school's assessment committee (typically a subcommittee of the curriculum committee) will have oversight of matters such as ensuring that the school's assessment policies are kept up to date, the timing and quantum of assessment, ensuring that the quality of assessment items is regularly reviewed and that faculty development is available to all those responsible for assessing students (see Fig. 4.2). Whenever the school changes its medical course, the assessment process and methods should reflect the changes in educational objectives.

Finally, not only should the standards and procedures for the assessment, advancement, and graduation be clear to all staff and students but also for disciplinary action. Each program should have in place a fair and formal process for taking any action that may affect the status of a medical student or trainee. This should include timely notice of any impending action, an opportunity to respond, and an opportunity to appeal any adverse decisions reached.

Summary
- Assessment in any medical education setting should reflect the educational objectives of the program and should be based on appropriate sampling of the program learning outcomes.
- A focus should be to provide high-quality formative assessment, through regular feedback.
- Assessment strategies should include direct observation of core clinical skills, behaviors, and the professional domains of practice.
- There should be a feasible assessment plan with a workload requirement that can be reasonably met by students and trainees.
- Faculty should have access to individuals with specific expertise in a variety of assessment formats.

References

1. Miller GE. The assessment of clinical skills/competence/performance. Acad Med. 1990;65(9 Suppl):S63–7.
2. Coderre S, Woloschuk W, McLaughlin K. Twelve tips for blueprinting. Med Teach. 2009;31(4):322–4.
3. Norcini JJ, Swanson DB, Grosso LJ, Shea JA, Webster GD. A comparison of knowledge, synthesis, and clinical judgment. Multiple-choice questions in the assessment of physician competence. Eval Health Prof. 1984;7(4):485–99 [Research Support, Non-U.S. Gov't].
4. Swanson DB, Holtzman KZ, Allbee K, Clauser BE. Psychometric characteristics and response times for content-parallel extended-matching and one-best-answer items in relation to number of options. Acad Med. 2006;81(10 Suppl):S52–5.
5. Page G, Bordage G, Allen T. Developing key-feature problems and examinations to assess clinical decision-making skills. Acad Med. 1995;70(3):194–201 [Research Support, Non-U.S. Gov't].
6. Feletti GI, Engel CE. The modified essay question for testing problem-solving skills. Med J Aust. 1980;1(2):79–80.

7. Harden RM. Twelve tips for organizing an Objective Structured Clinical Examination (OSCE). Med Teach. 1990;12(3–4): 259–64.

8. Friedman Ben David M, Davis MH, Harden RM, Howie PW, Ker J, Pippard MJ. AMEE Medical Education Guide No. 24: portfolios as a method of student assessment. Med Teach. 2001;23(6):535–51.

9. van der Vleuten CP. The assessment of professional competence: developments, research and practical implications. Adv Health Sci Educ. 1996;1(1):41–67.

10. Norcini J. Setting standards on educational tests. Med Educ. 2003;37(5):464–9.

11. van der Vleuten CP, Schuwirth LW. Assessing professional competence: from methods to programmes. Med Educ. 2005;39(3):309–17.

Chapter 5
Admission and Selection

Every medical education program should have an admission policy that specifies the requirements for entry into its program, that is, describe clearly the process used for *selecting* students and trainees. Typically, this information should be freely available on the program's website and in its published material. Such a policy should aim to minimize discrimination and bias and should address the mechanism available for appeals.

The admission policy should be cognizant of the health needs of the community in which the program operates. In the case of the medical school, the nature of the student cohort needs to be defined including quotas for students from underrepresented groups such as indigenous students and rural origin students. The school's admission policy should make clear the links between the selection process and the outcomes of the educational program. Typically, a central applications office manages all applications, and an accrediting team will be keen to examine the details of how this is done. For example, applicants may be assessed not just on results in secondary education but also on additional professional admissions tests [1, 2]. Where interviews are used, this will often be examined by a quality assurance team to ensure the process is as objective and fair as possible. Constructing an explicit structure and rating framework for the interviews can help achieve greater fairness and consistency.

G. MacCarrick, *Quality Assurance in Medical Education,*
DOI 10.1007/978-0-85729-713-6_5,
© Springer-Verlag London 2013

Typically, the responsibility for accepting students into a medical school rests with a medical school admissions committee; in some jurisdictions, this is a formally constituted committee with stipulated voting rights and community representation.

In terms of prerequisites for entry into medicine, some jurisdictions specifically encourage potential applicants to acquire a broad undergraduate education, including study of the humanities and the social sciences. This is increasingly the case with graduate entry medical programs citing the need for a broad-based undergraduate education as an important basis for the development of the ideal medical graduate. While there is no agreed method of selecting the most appropriate medical students into a medical school, an accrediting team will look for evidence of both academic and vocational considerations. In the case of selection for postgraduate training, the process should likewise be transparent and open to all qualified medical graduates. The criteria for selection may take into account factors such as ethnicity and a balanced gender intake. The language of instruction and the local health-care system are other considerations which need to be taken into account. For instance, fluency in written and spoken English may be a requirement for successful completion of the medical program, and the admission policy should reflect this. In all cases, the selection policy should be reviewed periodically, based on relevant societal and professional data to ensure the health needs of the community are being addressed.

Where part of the medical education takes place in rural or other locations, applicants should be advised accordingly. Information should be provided on the likelihood of this as well as how decisions regarding term allocations will be made.

In terms of the numbers of students or trainees a school/program enrolls, the size of the intake must reflect the capacity to deliver quality teaching and supervision. Student numbers and background should be reviewed in consultation with relevant stakeholders such as the teaching faculty and the clinical staff associated with the teaching hospitals and community clinics. In the postgraduate sector, trainee numbers should be derived in consultation with those responsible for medical manpower based on market and demographic forces as well as developments in health care. In some jurisdictions, publicly funded medical schools will have a predetermined domestic student intakes negotiated with government. Many medical schools also accept fee-paying or scholarship-supported students from other countries. If the medical school is an independent institution, it will have autonomy in setting its own student intake numbers each year.

While most medical education programs provide pathways for designated underrepresented groups, an accrediting team will be keen to see evidence of specific support mechanisms. In the case of basic medical education, this will include such resources as academic tutoring, cultural support (e.g., prayer rooms), counseling, mentoring, and physical facilities such as accommodation and financial support. In a similar way, students admitted from overseas, while they can enrich the educational experience for all students, should only be offered places if the quota does not exceed the school's capacity to deliver quality medical education. Appropriate language support for these students must be available. In addition, such students should be made aware on commencement of availability of access to local internships upon completion of training.

Support and Counseling

Support, including counseling, will be an important consideration when accrediting a medical education program. The well-being of medical students in particular as they make the adjustment to the physical and emotional demands of medical education needs to be taken into account. Typically, the medical school will have a welfare officer and/or a student support office, and students will have access to counseling and health services whether provided externally or by the medical school. It is important that students have the opportunity to seek support for any matter before it becomes a fitness to practice concern [3]. Some schools implement mentoring schemes or personal tutors as a way of supporting students. These roles should be made explicit to students. For instance, a medical student should have the option of obtaining advice about academic issues or counseling from individuals who do not participate in the assessment process. Opportunities should also exist for medical students who decide they are unsuited to medicine to exit the course early and receive counseling about further study and career options.

In the case of postgraduate training, trainees should also be provided with counseling services which address social and personal needs particularly around the time of making career decisions such as considering to change specialty programs.

In both basic and postgraduate medical education, quality assurance teams will examine how the program identifies and manages the poorly performing student and the trainee in difficulty. Often, the latter presents as failure to answer pagers, frequent lateness, excessive amounts of sick leave, and low work rate. A quality assurance team will be keen to examine what systems are in place for managing the under-performing trainee or student including what training is in place for mentors and tutors in this regard. Typically, this will include specific guidance on the conduct of face-to-face meetings and the documentation required (see Table 5.1).

TABLE 5.1 Example of record of meeting with trainee

Trainees name:	Date:
Meeting convened by:	
Current rotation:	
Purpose of meeting:	
Issues raised:	
Agreed action plan:	
Follow-up plan and date for next meeting:	

Increasingly medical schools are establishing "fitness to practice" committees in recognition of the fact that medical students have certain privileges and responsibilities which are different from those of other students requiring specific standards of professional behavior [3]. Breaches of these standards for health or behavioral reasons may compromise patient safety. While basic medical education should be able to accommodate a diverse student population including students with health conditions and disabilities, as well as different religious and cultural backgrounds, once graduated and entering the workforce, medical students must be fit to practice medicine. As such, the medical schools' fitness to practice committee will hear complaints or concerns raised about individual medical students. Typically, the committee will include a member from outside the medical school, a legal advisor, a student representative who does not know the student being investigated, and a registered medical professional. The role of the fitness to practice committee is to ensure proceedings are fair and comply with the legal requirements of equality and diversity.

As a critical stakeholder in the medical education process, students and trainees should have the opportunity to participate in the design, management, and evaluation of the program. Most medical schools will have a written policy on student representation on the relevant committees. Regular formal and informal meetings between faculty and students preferably with representation from all year levels will promote adequate exploration of student concerns and ensure input of student feedback and new ideas. Likewise, trainee representation on groups and committees responsible for program planning will ensure participation by trainees not only in program design, delivery, and evaluation but also participation in matters related to working conditions.

Student activities such as social clubs, sports groups, cultural clubs, etc. should be encouraged. A range of faculty and student-led initiatives will often improve integration particularly in schools where there is a wide range of cultural and ethnic backgrounds represented.

Quality assurance teams will explore policies relating to the admission of and procedures for the support of students with disabilities and students with infectious diseases, including blood-borne viruses. Health can adversely affect a student's fitness to practice, particularly when the problems have implications for the safety of patients or colleagues. It should be clear to such students how they will be accommodated in the medical course and what provisions can be made. Typically, this would include aspects such as physical accommodation for disabled students and support and counseling services for students with illness, impairment, and disability. With respect to students with infectious diseases, the policy should make explicit the school and the students' responsibility to ensure that patients are not put at risk from infected students. In addition, each school should have in place procedures for identifying and dealing with students with needs related to mental health or professional behavior issues. Policies and procedures on requirements for health records, immunizations, exposure to infectious agents or environmental hazards, insurance, and liability protection will often be examined by a quality assurance team. In some jurisdictions, student indebtedness is examined by accrediting teams including the average debt of current students as well as graduates, average scholarship support per student, and the percentage of total financial need supported by institutional and external grants and scholarships.

Summary Points
- The medical education program should have a publicly available transparent admission policy specifying the requirements for entry.
- The admission policy should make clear the links between the selection process and the outcomes of the educational program. The policy should be cognizant of the health needs of the community.

- The quality assurance team will look for evidence of both academic and vocational considerations in selecting students for entry.
- The target numbers of students or trainees should reflect the capacity to deliver quality teaching and supervision.
- Student/trainee support and counseling will be an important consideration when accrediting a medical education program.
- The program should have a clearly defined management plan for managing the underperforming trainee or student. Fitness to practice committees should ensure that proceedings are fair and compliant with the legal requirements of equality and diversity.

References

1. Coates H. Establishing the criterion validity of the Graduate Medical School Admissions Test (GAMSAT). Med Educ. 2008;42(10):999–1006 [Multicenter Study Research Support, Non-U.S. Gov't Validation Studies].
2. Powis DA. Selecting medical students. Med J Aust. 2008; 188(6):323–4.
3. General Medical Council G. Medical students: professional values and fitness to practise. General Medical Council. 2009. Available from: http://www.gmc-uk.org/education/undergraduate/professional_behaviour.asp. Cited Feb 2012.

Chapter 6
Medical School Resources

Faculty

A quality assurance team will examine the school's resources, that is, physical, human, and other assets that can be drawn on by the program to deliver its objectives and achieve its goal. An important aspect will be the sufficiency of the medical education program's teaching, research, and supervising faculty. In the case of the medical school, both the scientific and clinical disciplines will be reviewed to ensure the school has the capacity to meet the stated educational objectives of the program. Typically, each medical school will be expected to produce a detailed staff plan that outlines the type, responsibilities, and balance of academic staff required to deliver the curriculum (see Table 6.1). Such a plan will include the numbers of medical and nonmedical academic staff and the proportion of full-time to part-time staff. In the postgraduate training programs, the ratio of trainers to trainees should ensure sufficient interaction and support during the trainees' training period. Accrediting teams will need to be clear how much teaching time has been allocated to faculty particularly those with clinical or research responsibilities so that meaningful clinical teaching can occur across the continuum of medical education.

G. MacCarrick, *Quality Assurance in Medical Education,*
DOI 10.1007/978-0-85729-713-6_6,
© Springer-Verlag London 2013

TABLE 6.1 Example chart of school faculty numbers

Organizational unit	Academic staff	General staff	Total
Teaching:			
Medical education unit	2.6	2.3	4.9
Biomedical sciences program (year 1 and 2)	15.0		15.0
Intermediate program (year 3/4)	10.0		10.0
Clinical school A (year 5/6)	7.5		7.5
Clinical school B (year 5/6)	3.9	2	5.9
Rural clinical school (year 5/6)	3.8	3.7	7.5
Research:			
Research programs	10.7		10.7
Support services:			
Administrative services		13.2	13.2
Financial services		1.3	1.3
Research support services		1.5	1.5
Technical services		11.6	11.6
Total	*53.5*	*35.6*	*89.1*

The medical school human resource policies should include faculty appointments and how these are made, renewal of appointments, promotion, granting of tenure, indemnification, and dismissal. In terms of performance management typically all faculties would be expected to complete, in conjunction with their supervisor, a performance plan for each academic year. A feature of such a program would be linking this performance to the department and ultimately school's strategic plan. The supervisor reports on a staff member's performance, against his/her plan, and this is used in the assessment of promotion applications. In the postgraduate training sector, the human resource policies should stipulate the duties of trainers, the balance between training and service provision, and how trainers will be supported in their role. Typically, postgraduate trainers have a role in basic medical education and can avail of the faculty development offerings from both organizations, that is, university and college. It is important that each medical education program has clearly defined the responsibilities of its part-time hospital and community-based practitioners who contribute to the delivery of the medical course. Specifically, the medical school will have policies governing the awarding of honorary titles to medical practitioners and other health professionals who contribute to teaching.

In addition to teaching staff, there is a requirement for sufficient administrative and technical staff to support the educational program. Typically, administrative and technical staff are managed centrally in the medical school, thereby allowing the school to direct support as required. This model is also consistent with greater integration of the activities of the medical school avoiding discipline-based silos with departmentally based secretariat. The program's teaching and research effort require balanced administrative and technical support.

Academic staff need to have demonstrated academic achievements in his/her specialty area, and this should include demonstrated capacity and continued commitment to teaching as well as research. Individual faculty members should be able to present an accrediting team with evidence of participation in regular professional development activities related specifically to their discipline as well as their educator roles. This can be collated in the form of a teaching portfolio [4] (see Table 6.2). Typically, a teaching portfolio would contain specific details relating to teaching including long-term goals/objectives and how these might be attained. The coordination of the delivery of appropriate staff development in medical schools is the realm of Departments of Medical Education [1, 2]. The functions of such departments include research, teaching, and support of academic staff. Typically, such departments help staff acquire skills in large and small group teaching, student assessment, curriculum development and evaluation, and research in medical education. Based on the

TABLE 6.2 Example medical teacher portfolio

List of courses taught

Formal presentations, that is, lectures, tutorials, grand rounds, seminars delivered

Student results

Evaluation summaries (e.g., by peers, students)

Teaching awards and grants received

Medical school education committee involvement/position held

Positions held in national or international education committees/societies

Clinical supervisor/mentor responsibilities (students, junior doctors)

Curriculum and syllabus developed and role in this

List of Publications related to a curriculum/syllabus

List of Curriculum innovations and evaluation of these

Teaching materials published including videotapes/CD-ROMs/web-based teaching materials

current trends in medical education, some predict that formal medical education training will become compulsory for medical teachers in the future, suggesting that we can expect to see an increasing number of appointments made in specialized aspects of medical education, such as medical student assessment [3]. Albanese and colleagues found that a large number of medical education units were associated with the medical school dean's office and close communication with a supportive dean was an essential part of the successful medical education unit [1]. An accrediting team will also seek evidence of direct support and funding of the school's medical education unit.

As most medical schools will employ hospital and community-based practitioners to contribute to the delivery of the medical program, it is important that there exists a mechanism for communicating regularly its goals and objectives to these practitioners and includes this important cohort in the relevant faculty development offerings. Typical short courses include topics such as bedside clinical teaching, OSCE workshops, and item writing workshops. Some schools offer postgraduate taught programs (e.g., graduate certificate/ diploma and masters level programs in medical education), and some schools will subsidize attendance by staff to encourage participation. In addition, these programs can be "unbundled" to provide individual modules on specific topics of interest (for example, special modules on student assessment) which can also count toward continuing professional development of the medical practitioner. In addition to school-run programs, most universities offer formal taught programs for university teaching staff covering aspects including theoretical knowledge of how students learn and theoretical and practical knowledge about teaching, assessment, evaluation, and curriculum design. Such programs may also provide a useful resource particularly for new staff (see Table 6.3).

As the literature on medical education grows, medical students and postgraduate trainees are increasingly selecting research topics from this discipline. This will ultimately contribute to a larger pool of future academics with interest and expertise in the scholarship of teaching and learning.

All newly appointed academic staff, whether part-time or full-time, would typically be required to participate in a program which provides participants with the opportunity to expand their knowledge and skills and share experiences relating to their teaching practice. Most medical schools will have formal induction processes for new staff including written materials about the program. In addition, the medical school should have in place mechanisms for routinely evaluating all of its teacher effectiveness including clinical teachers at distant sites using feedback from students and other sources. In turn, individual faculty members should receive regularly scheduled feedback on his or her academic performance.

Ideally, the academic environment in which medical students and trainees learn should promote regular interaction between scientific and clinical staff in teaching, research, and health-care delivery. Regular fora focusing on aspects of the medical education program provides a useful strategy to

TABLE 6.3 Example table of contents for orientation manual – new staff

Campus parking information and map
Medical sciences building information
Key dates
Clinical academic appointments
Background to the curriculum
What is unique about our medical curriculum
The curriculum model and its five themes
Case-based learning in the new curriculum
Small group learning
The weekly timetable
Assessment
Role of the tutor
Role of the community placement supervisor
Mentoring
Teaching resources and support staff
Admin support
Library
WebCT Vista
Staff development and training opportunities

bring staff from different disciplines together to discuss areas of mutual educational interest.

Engaging with both undergraduate and postgraduate trainers at such events will promote greater integration across the educational continuum.

Educational Resources

An accrediting team will usually be interested in viewing some of the teaching sites to gauge whether there are sufficient physical facilities for students, trainees, and/or staff. Facilities inspected would typically include lecture theaters, tutorial rooms, laboratories, libraries, recreational facilities, examinations space, clinical skills facilities, small group teaching space, and additional student leisure facilities. It is rare that all sites can be viewed in what is typically a weeklong accreditation visit as distance between teaching sites can be significant. Focus will be on areas where changes have taken place or are proposed and matching stated educational objectives with physical resource. For example, schools that have embraced small group teaching need to have considered the need for adequate numbers of smaller-sized tutorial rooms which can be timetabled easily.

The medical school library plays an important role in most schools. The library not only provides access to electronic resources but increasingly supports the reference and information needs of all students, academic staff, research staff, and clinical academics. Many medical school libraries are also cognizant of space and function, library space being viewed increasingly as potential "learning spaces" – that is, multiuse, flexible use spaces equipped for small and large groups plus individual study space.

In terms of clinical teaching, each medical education program needs to ensure adequate exposure to primary, secondary, and tertiary care as well as ambulatory services, clinics, primary health-care settings, health-care centers, and other community health-care settings. As a consequence, the clinical training process tends to become dispersed across several teaching sites. The ensuing risk is that the quality of clinical teaching may become uneven and inconsistent across the sites. The objectives and assessment of clinical placements for both students and trainees need to be clearly defined and known to students, trainees, and staff. The program can monitor the fulfillment of the objectives of clinical placements in hospital and community teaching settings through regular site visits. Contractual agreements with the affiliated teaching hospitals and health service facilities should specify the contribution of clinical staff to teaching and supervision and the commitment expected by teaching staff to faculty development.

In terms of effective use of information and communication technology in the medical education program, staff and students should be encouraged and supported to use

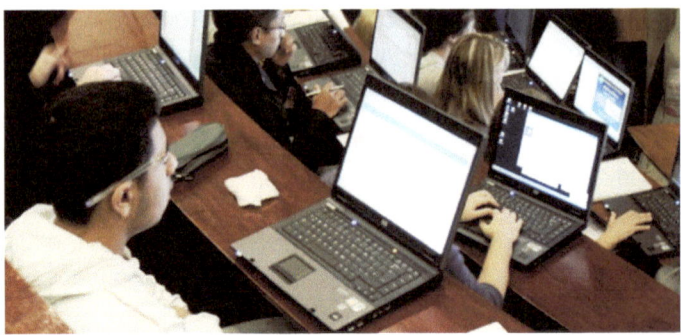

FIGURE 6.1 Information technology is significantly changing the way medical education is delivered

information and communication technology for self-learning, accessing information, managing patients, and working in health-care systems (see Fig. 6.1). Increasingly, information management systems are being utilized for many aspects of delivery and assessment of medical education programs requiring significant technical support staff. This is typically coordinated through a technical services unit. The program should aim to support a range of IT-related infrastructure and should remain committed to regularly evaluating information and communication technology used in the educational program. Some programs invest in a help desk arrangement for IT-related issues ensuring effective support to staff and students. System software and hardware should be regularly updated and standardized across all faculty computers. Library staff can be proactive in assisting both staff and students to be highly information literate by contributing to the delivery of programs on information-seeking skills. Students and trainees attending community-based attachments are typically exposed to the increasingly widespread use of clinical IT support systems at point of care. In recent years, hospitals have also seen increasing sophistication in IT systems, including pathology and radiology results retrieval, online incident reporting, and information resources on hospital intranet such as therapeutic guidelines. Students and trainees need to be exposed to these during their training. After hours, access to computer laboratories is also a consideration. A range of videoconference facilities typically support communication between sites when students or trainees are on rotation to rural settings. Wireless networks will further facilitate access to online resources.

Many programs have at their disposal increasingly sophisticated clinical skills laboratories in which students and trainees are able to develop basic and advanced clinical skills in a low-risk environment. How the program achieves a balance of simulated- and real-patient experience will be of particular interest to a quality assurance team.

Summary Points

- An important aspect of accreditation will be the program's resources, that is, physical, human, and other assets that can be drawn on by the program to deliver its objectives.
- The staff "profile" will be examined to ensure it is sufficient to deliver teaching, research, and supervision.
- All staff including hospital and community-based practitioners contributing to the delivery of the medical education program need to be familiar with the objectives of the program, adequately trained and supported in their educational role.
- Staff should have access to educational experts for the purpose of staff development and research.
- Facilities such as tutorial rooms, laboratories, clinical skills facilities, etc., should be sufficient to deliver and match the stated educational objectives of the program.
- Staff, students, and trainees should be supported in their use of information and communication technology for self-directed learning and managing patient care.

References

1. Albanese MA, Dottl S, et al. Offices of research in medical education: accomplishments and added value contributions. Teach Learn Med. 2001;13(4):258–67.
2. Davis MH, Karunathilake I, et al. AMEE Education Guide no. 28: the development and role of departments of medical education. Med Teach. 2005;27(8):665–75.
3. Harden RM. Editorial: building windmills not walls. Med Teach. 1998;20(3):189–91.
4. Tigelaar DE, Dolmans DH, et al. Participants' opinions on the usefulness of a teaching portfolio. Med Educ. 2006;40(4):371–8.

Chapter 7
Governance and Evaluation

Governance of the Program

A quality assurance process will examine the way in which the program is structured and how it functions as an organization. The program should make explicit the committee structure governing the activities of the program, and this should include appropriate representation from staff, trainers, students, and trainees. Relevant external stakeholders whose input should be sought would include medical councils, higher education authorities, national bodies responsible for medical workforce planning, and other representatives of the public and private health-care sector.

In the past, some of the barriers that faced curriculum committees included lack of administrative support to implement new ideas. A typical curricular governance structure of a medical school in the 1960s, for instance, was a curriculum committee composed of appointed or elected members representing the various school departments. Typically, there was no systematic evaluation of the course. Such departmental-based governance generated resistance to cross-disciplinary approaches and served only to reinforce departmental identity [5]. Most medical schools have now moved away from

G. MacCarrick, *Quality Assurance in Medical Education,*
DOI 10.1007/978-0-85729-713-6_7,
© Springer-Verlag London 2013

departmental-based governance to centralized governance, where the students' educational experience is organized around *what is taught,* not according to departmental structures and where there is a greater focus on continuous curriculum evaluation and renewal [6]. Quality assurance teams will be looking for evidence of governance that is consistent with the educational mission and objectives of the program.

Typically, the medical education program will have a central curriculum committee or board that has overarching responsibility to design and manage the medical curriculum (see Fig. 7.1). The accrediting team will be keen to see evidence of effective decision making by this committee and sufficient authority and autonomy to make necessary curriculum changes. Appropriate budgetary responsibility and accountability should accompany the governance structures. This board will typically have reporting it to its various subcommittees responsible for particular aspects of the curriculum such as assessment and evaluation.

Governance arrangements should ensure sufficient autonomy and control over the decisions including the program's overall strategic direction, budget allocation and expenditure, development of new courses, and staff appointments. Each of the committee's terms of reference and membership should be clearly articulated. Faculty should have full access to committee meeting agendas and minutes, and there should be evidence of wide dissemination of draft policies and procedures for faculty members' input.

The highest level of authority within the medical education program should aspire to promote an environment of academic excellence under which teaching and research can flourish.

A key challenge will be to ensure that the ambitions of the program's lead academic (e.g., the medical school dean or college chief executive) are resourced appropriately and supported to allow for the implementation of innovation. Understanding of the various leadership and governance styles necessary to lead support and sustain medical education programs is critical. Several studies have looked at leadership styles in medical education. Participative leadership

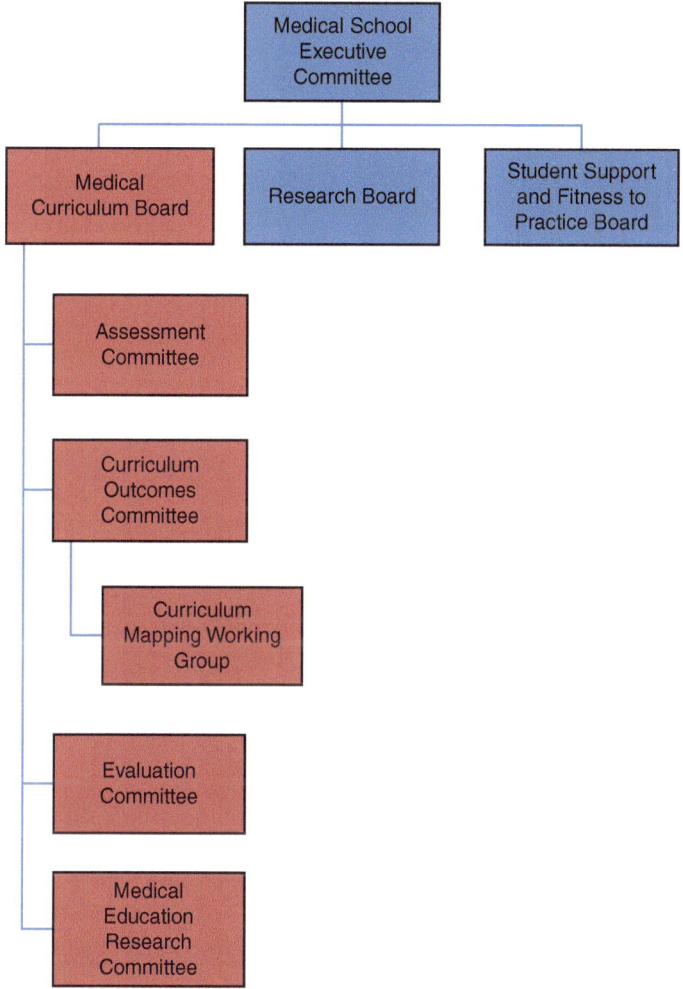

FIGURE 7.1 Example medical school governance structures

behaviors were more likely to be correlated with successful achievement of desired curriculum reforms [1, 2]. The literature also acknowledges the different styles required for different occasions. For instance, leading a medical school through a period of significant curriculum reform requires a different type of leadership than that required when the school is undergoing a more stable time in its history. A quality assurance team will be keen to see that the responsibilities of the academic leadership of the medical educational program are clearly stated and evaluated at defined intervals with respect to achievement of the mission and objectives of the program. Most programs recognize the risk that educational leadership will lack focus and drive unless a senior post is created heading the educational development dimensions. In most medical schools, this position is filled by a Director of Medical Education. Such individuals lead the curriculum reform efforts through chairing the various committees charged with developing new aspects of the curriculum. This individual must be well supported financially by the dean and is typically selected based on his/her ability to lead curriculum change. Recognizing that in most medical schools, such a person is usually appointed as an associate dean, and therefore subordinate to the dean the relevant operational authority issues need to be addressed. Communication between the dean and the associate dean is essential such that together they can communicate effectively the vision for the program's future.

In addition to academic leadership, the administrative staff of the medical school must be appropriate to support the implementation of the school's educational program and other activities and to ensure good management and deployment of its resources.

Engagement with Stakeholders in the Health Sector

All medical education programs should aim to establish a constructive interaction with the health and health-related sectors of society and government. This would typically include public and private hospitals, departments of health, medical research institutions, regulating bodies, health promotion, and public policy organizations. The level of demand on the dean of the

TABLE 7.1 Example membership of medical school advisory committee

Department of Health and Human Services	Director (Chair)
University	Deputy vice-chancellor Dean
Medical association	President
Medical council	President
College of Anaesthetists	Nominee
College for Emergency Medicine	Nominee
College of General Practitioners	Nominee
College of Obstetricians and Gynaecologists	Nominee
College of Ophthalmologists	Nominee
Association of Orthopaedics	Nominee
College of Physicians	Nominee
College of Surgeons	Nominee

medical school, for example, in dealing with the complexities of the interactions with the health sector, can be significant. Key among the partnerships the dean would seek to support are those with public and private hospitals as well as community-based health-care facilities which provide clinical placements for students and/or trainees. Many of these relationships are protected using Memorandums of Understanding.

Agreements between departments of health and medical schools for instance can ensure better collaboration to improve health services for the community and address the increasing demands being placed on the health-care system. Some medical schools establish advisory committees to act as an external stakeholder committee (see Table 7.1). Typically, this provides a forum through which its members, mainly representatives of the branches of the various medical colleges and associations, can provide support, assistance, and advice to the dean on matters affecting the ongoing activities and future of the school.

Specialist medical colleges likewise provide training in complex environments influenced by health policies, legislation, and structures of multiple jurisdictions. Issues around the environment for training and teaching require college and jurisdictional cooperation. Competition between service demands and training impacts upon training and teaching; hence, partnerships between postgraduate medical training programs and various jurisdictions can ensure both a safe working environment and a training program that produces medical specialists capable of meeting the needs of the community. Such statements of mutual intent can, for example, agree to support clinical and professional education with personnel and infrastructure across the learning continuum; appoint and develop faculty to provide quality teaching, research, and clinical service delivery; support research that informs and supports service delivery, teaching, and workforce development; and develop reform models to build a flexible, sustainable health system.

Evaluating the Program

Society has a keen interest in how doctors are trained and in ensuring that medical schools and postgraduate training programs produce graduates who are capable of fulfilling the needs of the community. Ongoing program evaluation therefore plays a key role in all activities of any curriculum, particularly a curriculum where the underlying knowledge base is increasing exponentially as is the case with medicine.

Evaluation in medical education includes a whole range of methods, the primary goal of which is to provide useful information to guide and improve programs and assist decision makers. Evaluation of the outcomes of medical education is a complex area not the least because of the time lapse between the educational intervention and the overall result, that is, successful performance as an independent medical practitioner. To simply collect evaluation data is not good enough. Information gained should guide program planning and activities. The purpose of the evaluation strategy should be to ensure continuous improvement of the quality and outcomes of the medical education program. Key principles underpinning any evaluation strategy include evaluation that is ongoing, meaningful, timely, relevant, credible, objective, affordable, and ethical. Evaluation should address the specific components of the curriculum such as course content and student performance and the general outcome of the program as measured for instance by career choice and postgraduate performance (see Table 7.2).

Typically, the medical education program will evaluate content such as modules, units, or rotations of the program on a "rolling" cycle (see Table 7.3). Central coordination of evaluation will ensure standardized processes are in place and will ensure feedback from data collected is distributed widely. A quality assurance team will be keen to examine the types of evaluation tools used such as web-based surveys and focus groups, etc. It is important that the information gained is communicated back to students and staff, that is, the evaluation loop is closed.

Some programs invest in tracking and surveys of recent graduates or alumni.

Tracking studies typically require significant investment of time but provide valuable data about graduate career choice and contribution to the workforce [3]. Graduate surveys can invite recent graduates to comment on their preparedness for

TABLE 7.2 Example terms of reference of medical school evaluation committee

The evaluation committee will:
Provide the central coordination of all curriculum evaluation activities
Prepare the annual evaluation work plan on behalf of the medical education committee
Ensure the progress of ongoing evaluation is reported to medical education committee on a monthly basis
Ensure evaluation strategies are incorporated into new and developing curriculum initiatives
Maintain an up-to-date database of all curriculum evaluation activities

TABLE 7.3 Example questionnaire used to survey student satisfaction with tutorials

Do you agree or disagree with the following statements:	1 Disagree strongly	2 Disagree	3 Neutral	4 Agree	5 Agree strongly	Mean rating
Were clearly linked to the lecture series	1	8	35	52	4	3.5
Assisted me in my understanding the lecture	1	15	42	40	2	3.3
Were a positive experience for me	1	12	41	41	5	3.4
My tutor:						
Encouraged everyone to actively participate	—	3	23	67	8	3.8
Responded to questions effectively	—	1	27	62	9	3.8
Encouraged me to extend my thinking about the subject matter	1	5	34	52	9	3.6
Showed interest in my learning	1	5	48	43	4	3.4

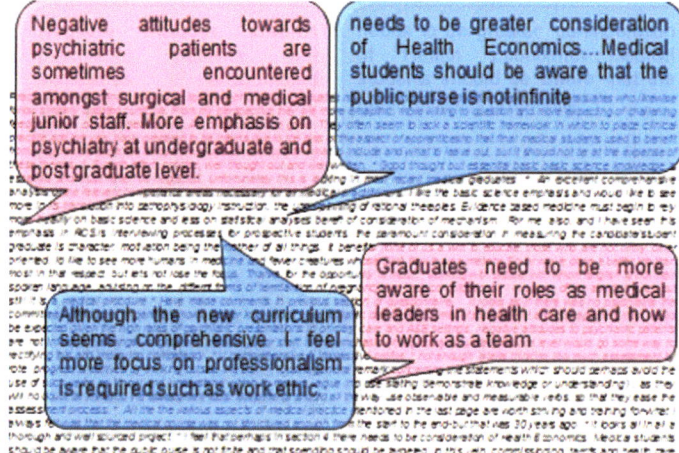

FIGURE 7.2 Feedback from alumni can inform ongoing curriculum renewal

hospital practice [4] or ask for feedback about the curriculum or proposed curriculum reforms. Accreditation teams will be keen to see that the information gathered from current students, trainees, and graduates of the program is used to inform the subsequent development and design of the curriculum including revision as necessary of curriculum outcomes, delivery methods used, and assessment of student/trainee learning (see Fig. 7.2).

It is critical that faculty, students, and trainees be active members of the program evaluation process with a transparent mechanism for analyzing the results of all evaluations conducted. There should be broad representation of all the committees which collect evaluation data (see Table 7.4). In particular, student or trainee representation will ensure the design of instruments of program evaluation is relevant and understood. An appreciation of the views, experiences, and needs of faculty, including clinical teachers in the partner hospitals, should be captured as part of the evaluation process.

An important factor in planning new evaluation strategies will be to consider the burden of evaluation on students or

TABLE 7.4 Example membership of a medical school evaluation committee

Independent chair (appointed by the dean)
Industry advisory body representative – member of the school of medicine advisory committee
Representative of accrediting body (e.g., medical council)
Representative of the Department of Health
Pro-vice-chancellor (teaching and learning), university
Representative of Committee of Deans of Medical Schools
Representative of Postgraduate Medical Council
Representative medical students including international students
Consumer representative, for example, Patient Advocacy Group

trainees. Faculty are often keen to evaluate new modules or new innovation and however need to be cognizant that "overevaluation" is avoided, which can lead to deterioration of the quality of the data gathered.

The performance of cohorts of students or trainees is an important aspect of program evaluation. Performance data such as pass rates and attrition rates should be analyzed in relation to student/trainee background and entrance qualifications. Such information can be used to provide feedback to the program's selection committees as well as committees responsible for support and counseling (see Fig. 7.3). The results of program evaluation should ideally be made available to the widest possible stakeholder group.

Such a group would include representatives of the community, professional organizations, and those responsible for undergraduate and postgraduate education. The engagement of this key external stakeholders group is critical to the success of the curriculum renewal processes such as redrafting curriculum outcomes and maintaining alignment with changes to health-care practice. A dynamic medical education program will have procedures in place to continually review its activities to ensure the program remains responsive to changes in health care and new developments in education.

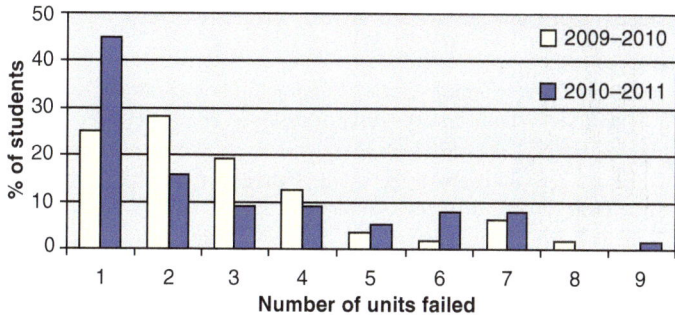

FIGURE 7.3 Performance data can assist curriculum design and inform selection/entry criteria

Summary Points

- The medical education program should make explicit the committee structures governing the activities of the program and this should include appropriate representation from students or trainees.
- Governance needs to reflect the educational missions and objectives of the program and should ensure autonomy and control over the decision making including the program's overall strategic direction and budget allocation.
- The responsibilities of the academic leadership of the program should be made clear.
- All medical education programs should aim to establish a constructive interaction with other health-related stakeholders and the communities they serve.
- Program Evaluation should be transparent and address the content and context of the curriculum and the outcome of the program.
- Accreditation teams will be keen to see that feedback about the program is used to inform subsequent development and design.

References

1. Bland CJ, Starnaman S, et al. Leadership behaviors for successful university – community collaborations to change curricula. Acad Med. 1999;74(11):1227–37.
2. Bland CJ, Starnaman S, et al. Curricular change in medical schools: how to succeed. Acad Med. 2000;75(6):575–94.
3. Harris MG, Gavel PH, et al. Factors influencing the choice of specialty of Australian medical graduates. Med J Aust. 2005;183(6):295–300.
4. Hill J, Rolfe IE, et al. Do junior doctors feel they are prepared for hospital practice? A study of graduates from traditional and non-traditional medical schools. Med Educ. 1998;32(1):19–24.
5. Reynolds 3rd CF, Adler S, et al. The undergraduate medical curriculum: centralized versus departmentalized. Acad Med. 1995;70(8):671–5.
6. Davis W, White C. Managing the Curriculum and Managing Change. In: Norman GR, van der Vleuten CPM, Newble DI, editors. International Handbook of Research in Medical Education: Kluwer Academic Publishers; 2002. p. 917–44.

Index